DROP THE
BAGGAGE

From Suicidal Obesity to a Life of Health and Happiness

DAVID RODEN

ACKNOWLEDGMENTS

To the most incredible family, a man can ask for, my love and gratefulness to you all will always be the driving force in everything I do.

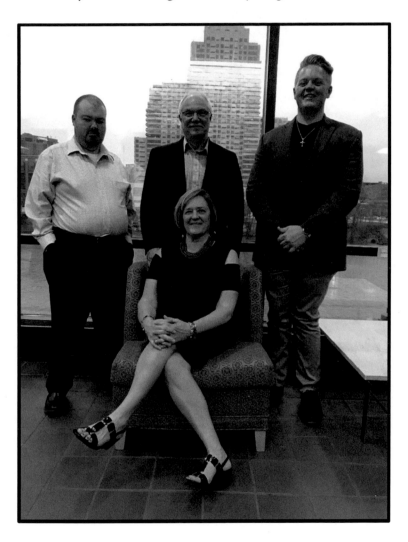

Table of Contents

INTRODUCTION

First and foremost, thank you so much for purchasing my book. I am beyond excited for you to take in the habits and experiences I have used over the last 5+ years of my life and utilize the information to create a drastic shift in yours. I feel beyond blessed you took time and money out of your life to learn from me.

Before I go into depths on my story and information, I will give you that thumbnail sketch from where I came from to where I am at in this current day. Sitting here in my room writing this. To even think I would be writing a book on how to transform your mind and body is wild in multiple ways. First I told myself for YEARS I was not a reader or a writer. I did not read a book cover to cover till around Junior year of COLLEGE! I told myself a false story that I was not a reader or writer because I was in slow reading classes when I was in third and fourth grade. I told myself that story all the way till JUNIOR YEAR OF COLLEGE! What fake stories are you telling yourself because of some past event from your childhood?

Also, to be writing a book on how to build YOUR IDEAL body from a kid who was over 400 pounds by the time I was 18 years old! Pre Diabetic, I took Metformin for my increase in insulin sensitivity. My resting blood pressure without medication was 190/120. I could not hold a jog on the track at school for just the straightaway. When we did the fitness tests in High School, I failed all of them except for the Sit and Reach! I would sit and play videos games for HOURS each day. Fast forward to today I have lost over 160 pounds SUSTAINABLY. I am off ALL of my medications.

Now, in the process of bodybuilding to a YOLKED 6pack piece of MAN MEAT! Writing this book on how you can do it too! I am not unique or any different than you reading this. I actually was probably in a worse situation mentally because not only was I so OBESE and POOR MENTALLY but I had such a fortunate upbringing. My father is a Cardiologist, and I was very knowledgeable about how the body works. So I couldn't play on the ignorance of "not knowing." I knew exactly what I was doing to myself and felt helpless about how to change it. I wouldn't change my past struggles for anything. It has made me into who I am today. You WILL get to that point too. Make your battles DEFINE you, not DEFEAT you.

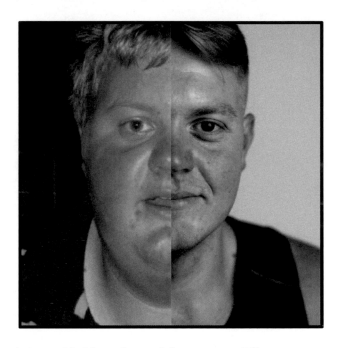

With that being said, I have learned from many different mentors over the years. Utilizing knowledge and ideas from Tony Robbins, Les Brown, Kevin Trudeau, Napoleon Hill, Jesus, Jim Rohn, Tim Ferris and many many more. Throughout this book, I will do my best to give credit where credit is due. Most of this information is not my own, but the knowledge I have learned and utilized in my own life. This book will be focused on how to create a drastic shift in your MIND and BODY. I will be sharing foundational information on how to create the HABITS and DECISIONS you "WANT" to make but haven't seemed to be able to do. Some people will find this book as "entertainment," meaning that they will just read it and be like, "oh wow, very inspiring stuff." Others will throughout the book take notes and highlight certain parts that resonate with them, but will never read over what they emphasized. Then there will be another group who will underline and take notes. Read over those notes and will see how they can implement pieces of the book into their own lives. Also, after a certain amount of time reread their notes and highlights to see how they are doing. I will also be making it easier to you to take notes because I will be leaving blank lines and activities to do to help use more of your mental capacity by not just READING but also WRITING and SPEAKING. As you do these activities, depending on where you are in your journey, these activities may come easily to you and also may be very difficult. Now, don't skip the activities, take your time with them. Use as much time and effort you can to really dig deep. The more mental energy you use during these exercises, the more impact you will have on yourself. With that being said, every activity you will do is something I have done on myself over the last 5 years that have helped create the DRASTIC growth in my life.

Now I want to set up some expectations for you while you read. The first thing to know is that 90% of people who read a book on personal growth and achievement never read past the first chapter. So I challenge you to read this in its entirety. Hold to an agreement to yourself that you will utilize 1-3 ideas in this to take ACTION on in your own life. We have all been told that "KNOWLEDGE IS POWER" and sadly that is not the case. "THE STORAGE AND EFFECTIVE USE OF KNOWLEDGE IS POWER." If knowledge were power, you would already have your IDEAL body and be living the life you truly want. However, that is not the case because we miss the implementation of information into our daily lives. We all know eating leafy greens and salads are better than eating double stuffed fried Twinkie's. We all understand that you should be drinking less sugar-filled pop and more water. You have that "Knowledge," but you are not acting on it. That is one of the most significant issues you are having to this day. Turning KNOWLEDGE into ACTION. So throughout this book, take notes! Write solid plans of ACTION you are going to bring in your own life. You will be blown away by just using a few simple ideas in this book can and will make a DRASTIC shift in your life.

There is no question that if you are reading this, you have at least the little piece of you that is ready for CHANGE! No one would even be reading this book if they did not have at least a portion of them prepared for change. For most people, you will never have the clouds open up, and God says to you with angels singing, "IT'S TIME MY CHILD." You take it day by day. Moment by moment you build momentum into positive change in your life. So are you ready? Are you prepared to make HUGE GROWTH!? Well, I am EXCITED for you!

This book is not about giving you some cookie cutter way to lose some weight. The intention behind this book is to share with you the basics needed to take 100% control over your life and your body. Through reading this book, I want to give you the basic understanding to FOREVER be in control of your life with all of the possibilities available to you. You have the opportunity with this book to recreate your destiny. Recreate what it means to be you. Recreate what your IDEAL body looks like. Give you different options and plans that can work for you and see if they are the right fit for you. There is no one size fits all nutrition plan. You must know the foundation to nutrition and what possible plans there are out there and why they work and who they work for. All of the nutrition plans I will be discussing I have used and have worked for me in my journey.

In comparison to your body, there are very few things with such a few amounts of elements that make up a strong and stable body compared to a weak, erratic one. Taking 100% responsibility for your body is an absolute must, no matter the circumstances.

There are countless stories of people going above the odds to take 100% responsibility for their life, regardless of their circumstances. We are really drawn to it as people. Watching people go above and beyond what is expected of them to do something extraordinary. Have you ever seen a movie of someone doing something average or normal?

One of my favorites is the story of Ben Mudge. Ben was diagnosed with degenerative lung disease from birth known as Cystic Fibrosis. Cystic Fibrosis, if you are unaware, is indeed a death sentence. It is a condition where your lungs begin to fill with thick mucus that slowly fills the lungs over time, till you can no longer breathe. There is no cure. However, even with this diagnosis, he took 100% responsibility for his body and his life. Knowing how good exercise is for a person like him. Activity, moving air in and out of his lungs at high pressure and volume kept his mucous lower. So he took this to the extreme because in his situation he had to. His incentive to working out meant living. So he worked out with big compound movements 5-7 times a week for at least an hour. That intense training regiment kept the mucous down. One of the by-products of his intense workout schedule was a "Thor Like" body. He is now very sculpted in his physique. Ben could have quickly fallen into the victim trap. Blaming and pointing fingers at everything. What he was going through was unfair, but he dared to take 100% responsibility, regardless of making the best out of his situation. No matter what you are going through, you have that opportunity today.

I challenge you to be HONEST with yourself. You expect others to be HONEST with you. How HONEST are you with yourself? We lie to ourselves so often. Often enough where we barely notice we are anymore. This book will create ten times more impact if throughout this you are TRULY HONEST with yourself. How are you feeling? What fears are you dealing with? The struggles you are having? Your strengths. Your weaknesses. The lies you are telling yourself to keep you safe are really holding you back.

CHAPTER 1

My story up till now

To really understand how "normal" I am; I would love to share my complete story. Growing up in Grand Rapids, Michigan, I was born into a very blessed family. My mother is one of the most supportive giving people you will ever meet. From always putting on school parties to taking in my friends when they either had tough family upbringings or just for extra support. She was always there to pick me up or take me anywhere. My father, as I stated before is a cardiologist. Also known as a heart doctor. He grew up on the south side of Chicago. Giving him a great perspective of what growing up with less was like. I went to Forest Hills school district. Forest Hills was a great affluent school district but what also gave me great pleasure was going to Northern because it had some of the most diverse student body of the district. I was always the outgoing kid with more friends than I had time in a day for. When walking the neighborhood as a child, my parents would hear from the neighbors, "oh you are David's parents." Meaning I loved to talk to new people and have a fun conversation from a very early age. For pretty much my entire childhood all I can remember is being overweight. I, like many others, was bullied and called fat. Now at the same time looking back, no one could bully me as much I was bullying myself. As I hit High School, I was over 300 pounds. In that time I was 13-14 already on blood pressure meds and pre-diabetic meds. On the outside, I had it all together. The "smart" and "funny fat kid" but on the inside, I was in a silent state of desperation.

I am asked over and over again if you had such a great supportive family, how did you get so obese? It really is simple. Growing up my mom wanted to make sure I felt fully loved. In her eyes making sure I felt fully loved meant to always say yes to what I wanted. As a kid with pretty much-unlimited money and support, what did I want? FOOD!! So as I grew up, I became INFATUATED with food. I loved food and loved the full feeling I got after I ate. Now, what did I eat? You will laugh. I was drinking 15-20 diet cokes a day. Drinking so many a day that when I would ask Phil, my best friend from High School, to go get me a few more, he would say no, and he would not support the bad habit. I loved diet coke so much that I almost talked my dad into getting a fountain diet coke machine in the house because it would save him money. I would also eat an entire Costco size bag of Reese's like 18-24 Reese's a day. I would hide the wrappers in the bottom drawer next to my tv then every few days I would bring the pile of wrappers to the trash and make sure I shoved them to the bottom, so mom and dad did not see.

I LOOOOOVED food. All food. Eat an entire large Jets pizza to myself. Late night Taco Bell or McDonald's runs at 12am-2am would also happen multiple times a week. We are not talking like a 6-7 dollar meal. I would drop 15-20 dollars in food from McDonald's or Taco Bell. We all know that is ALOT of food. I was also a HUUUUGE gamer. Staying up late to play Call of Duty or World of Warcraft till 2,3, even 4 am. I could sit in my computer chair for multiple hours having sugar rushes due to all of the candy and pop. Still playing away. So you add that up. Poor eating habits + never told no + sedentary lifestyle = FATTTT

In High School, I did "try" multiple times to lose weight. The generic way that we all try. I see an infomercial on _____ plan on either nutrition or workout plans. With the love and support of my family, they ALWAYS gave me any program under the sun. I had the Ab Lounger. I did that for a whole 2-3 days. Then after I saw I commercial on P90x and was like…. "YES! That's it!" So a week later I was a Tony Horton guy doing P90x for a few weeks. Then quit that bad boy. Next was the Bowflex. And so on…… and so on…. and so on….. I went through MULTIPLE programs in High School. What is also interesting is how I created a story about why I was overweight.

As you have seen from my earlier story, I shared with you how I ate and treated my body. As are you justifying or rationalizing your weight. I had a cyst, or growth, on my brain. The growth was on my pituitary gland. This gland affects a lot of your metabolic systems. So for about a 2 year time, I had to get brain scans to see if it ever got bigger to reevaluate what we needed to do. I had multiple doctors tell me, "this could be the reason why you are overweight." One of my doctors had made the statement we could put you in the desert for a few months, and you may not lose weight. Hearing this allowed me to justify my habits. Your desire to eat and drink is not your fault. It is something out of your control. However, when you really think about it, you know that really isn't true. Thank God after 2 years the growth just went away. However, I still would use that excuse.

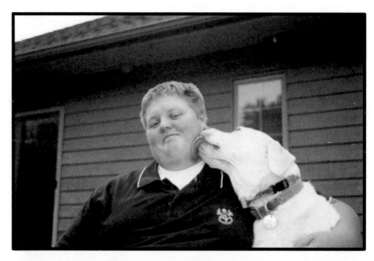

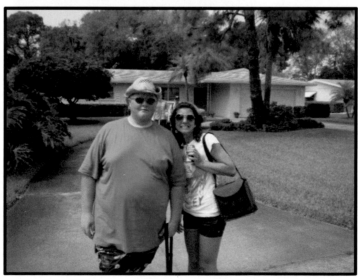

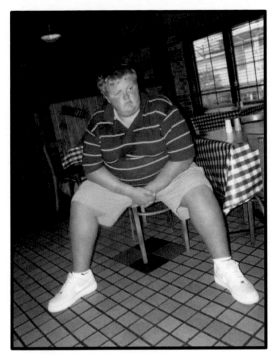

Not only was my body in such poor habits but also my mind. This is where my story in my mind gets fascinating. Longterm in my life this is where I want to go with my story. To fill in more depths of how blessed I was growing up, I'll add a few more details. I grew up in a 7,000+ square foot house with an indoor basketball court. I had 5 cleaning ladies go through the house every other week to change my sheets and do EVERYTHING. My mother literally would do ANYTHING I ask to help support me. Giving me her credit card to go to movies and dinner with all of my friends and I paid for it all. I still remember to this day when I was young my dad had me stand on the sink in the bathroom while he shaved. He would tell me, "Hey David, look at that man across from you, tell him you love him." Always giving me love and support. The idea that I can BE DO or HAVE anything I want in this world. They never pushed me into any field or what I should do with my life. I truly NEVER heard my parents argue as a kid. So you look at my upbringing. You would probably say I had the IDEAL childhood. All the resources. All of the support. All of the love. Most people think that some RESOURCE is holding them back from success and happiness. I HAD IT ALL! At the same time, I can VIVIDLY remember me laying in my shower crying my eyes out. Hold scissors to my wrists trying to build the courage to end my life. I WANTED TO KILL MYSELF! You know how people make the general line of, "YOU CREATE YOUR OWN REALITY." It is more real than you know. I think the most significant opportunity for experience is not seeing someone doing it right but doing it so wrong it's obvious. I created a reality in my own head that…I was worthless… I would NEVER amount to anything… I was too far gone… I am a failure… I will never aspire to the level of success I should have because of my family is expecting… My grades were plummeting my junior-senior of High school. For friends and family, the last paragraph may come to a shock to you. For the fact that on the outside it looked like I had it all together. I believe most of us are a lot better at hiding where our emotions are really at. To think the kid with all the friends all the family and all the resources you could ask for almost killed himself twice shows you that you can REALLLLY mess up how your mind works. Now with that being said, I am so excited to share with you some of the fundamentals to how the mind works to BECOME the INSPIRED ALWAYS HAPPY guy you see today. It's not some HOGY mantra of meditations and speeches but a solid understanding of your emotional and physical struggles and what you have been doing wrong and how to fix it.

Thank God I didn't follow through with my suicidal thoughts. After High School, I went to Central Michigan University. Where I studied biology with a focus in medicine. I was blessed to have randomly been placed in a room with a few awesome guys. This was the first time I was on my own. Where you can, "reevaluate your life." Your environment overnight completely changes. Even though it varies depending on where you are it may not change much. One of my roommates Troy was a High School runner but also a gamer. Which made a high starting point for me. We were able to game often but also started the initial momentum of trying to get my body more in order. Halfway into freshman year, he made a bet with me that I couldn't work out for 30 days straight. Now it's up for discussion if I won the bet or not because I got sick one of the days sooooo I say I won, but he says I didn't.

What is more important is what I learned. As I would work out for the 30 days, I went straight into weight training. In my personal opinion, someone as out of shape as I was should acclimate your body to the changes ahead. I would wake up with such bad cramps while I was sleeping that I would

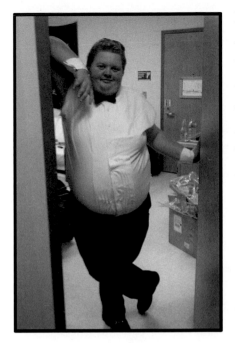

literally scream and cry from the pain. My quads and hamstrings got so tight that it felt like my leg was going to snap in half. I would be in the middle of playing Call of Duty with troy, and my arms would cramp up, and I would drop the controller. He laughed hysterically. What I took from the experience is that for anyone in the morbidly obese stage should not start with strength training. It is important in the long term of a healthy body but when you are that out of shape just getting the body moving is so important. Otherwise, most people when they hit the massive cramps stage will stop. Just like I did. I found that pain not worth the change at the time.

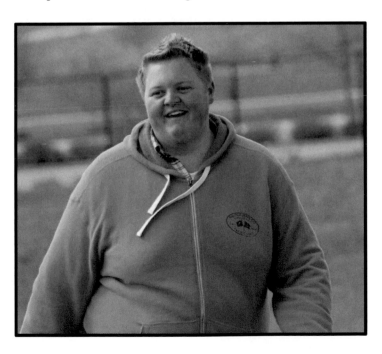

The big transition in my life happened in my third year of college. During this time I was getting towards the later part of my college career. Knowing I needed to start thinking long and hard about what I wanted to do after college. I looked at the idea of being a doctor. So I looked at my dad's life as a reference. I loved the income and resources available when you are a doctor. However, I was not too enthused on the hours and lack of control over your hours as a doctor. When my dad was at his peak of workload. He would work on-call and weekends multiple times a year. On an average week, my dad would easily put in 50-70 hours between the hospital and the office. When he would have to work on-call and weekends, he could push 90 hours. That was something that I did not want. While I was questioning what I wanted to do, my father also wanted me to become more self-sufficient, so he insisted I look to make an income. At this time we have all experienced those Facebook messages or texts saying, "I HAVE AN OPPORTUNITY OF A LIFETIME!! YOU HAVE TO CHECK IT OUT". Coming from money I was often asked to borrow money or invest in something. Now, I do still respect people's time and information, so I sat down with my buddy Brandon. He shared with me this company called VEMMA. It was a health and nutrition company using the Network Marketing strategy for sales. Growing up in Grand Rapids I knew what Network Marketing was on a basic level. Between family in other companies and Amway world headquarters was down the street from I knew it was something. After my first sit down with Brandon, I got on the phone with a great guy, Scotty. We-vibe heavy just on where we were in life. What we wanted and how the system was set up for money and success. I knew after that convo that I may like this. Lose weight on some cool weight loss products and make money while doing it? Sounds good to me. I drove down to East Lansing and met a few kids that would TRANSFORM my life FOREVER! At the time I had asked my dad what he thought about the products and opportunity and gave me his positive outlook of, "if you are willing to work hard for it do it." So at that point, I joined VEMMA and begin the most significant transformation in my life.

At this time I began to read books on self-improvement and personal growth. Luke and Jamie gave me different books that helped them. It's amazing how your own life changes when you surround yourself with different people. This new group of friends had an expectation in their group for personal growth. The first book I was recommended was, The Compound Affect by Darren Hardy. Up to this point in my life, I had never read a book cover to cover. I use to spark note or sneak by with my natural intelligence. This book was the first book that gave me the idea of how life really works. How the success and failures in life don't come from these HUGE DECISIONS of "do I go to Central Michigan University or Michigan State University?", "Do I do the KETO diet or MACRO COUNTING?". Your success and failures in life are more determined by the almost unnoticed decisions of….. "Do I eat a salad or a pizza?"…. "Do I workout or sleep in?"….. "Do I read or do I play video games?"… These almost unnoticeable decisions compounded over a long period to make a more real impact on your life than the HUGE DECISIONS we tend to only focus on. Also, it gave me the power to understand that if you just change a few simple habits over an extended time that a HUGE CHANGE will happen. There are 3500 calories in a pound. So thinking about the idea of losing 200 pounds sounds so far out of reach but when you break it down to knowing there are 3500 calories in a pound. I want to lose 2 pounds a week. That's 8 pounds a month. Which is 96 pounds a year. That means in 2 years of cutting 7,000 calories a week from working out and eating better, you WILL hit your goal! Wow! Ok, let's break down the week and day. Wow, if I eat 4 meals of BLANK nutrition and workout BLANK amount of time a day. Over a week time, I burn 7000 more calories a week than I take in. Compound that over 2 years I HIT MY GOAL! I can do that. Chunking down your goal into more bite-size pieces will compound out to your ULTIMATE GOAL! I can do that.

When it comes to the DRASTIC TRANSFORMATION that I created over the next few years in VEMMA came down to 4 foundational pieces. I began to read daily. Reading each and everyday charges and primes your mind into learning information. However, as I read, I made sure to take pieces of what I was reading to utilize in my everyday life. I would read for 30 minutes EVERY DAY. I made it a daily habit just like brushing my teeth. Next, I made sure that I turned my car into a mobile classroom. Going into my final year at CMU I was taking 19 credit hours of 300+ level bio and chemistry classes. I did not have a lot of time to put into learning outside of school. So while I would drive to class or anywhere, I began to listen to audios. Speeches or audio books on different information. This gave me a new NET time I didn't have to learn continually. NET time is also known as NO EXTRA TIME. We all think we have a "full schedule." I utilized time that I was not efficiently using into more intentional time.

Learning while in the car driving to school and other activities gave me that extra time needed to keep my mind on keeping my momentum of growth of success in my habits going. The next action that was added was weekly events with other like-minded people in that wanted the same things out of life. These small events would RECHARGE my battery giving me the ENERGY and FOCUS to keep me going. Finally, I would go to a YEARY or BI YEARLY event that would put me into a full emersion of NEW INFORMATION and HIGH ENERGY that created such EMOTIONAL IMPACT that it would help keep my drive at 100%. These 4 basics are VITAL to keeping your momentum going in your transformation. Start reading EVERY DAY! Even if only 5 pages.

Listen to something EVERYDAY. Use either an audiobook or Youtube to hear from people to learn from. Next, find a small group of people you can meet up with weekly that are focusing on the same things you are. This could be a gym group or networking group. Finally, go to at least once a year a BIG EVENT to EMERSE yourself in new information at a HIGH ENERGY LEVEL to help create EMOTIONAL IMPACT. Some ideas could be Tony Robbins events, Fitness events, Network Marketing Events. Some large group with HIGH ENERGY to RECHARGE and help you have a substantial EMOTIONAL IMPACT. I still do all these to this day.

For three years I was building and growing with VEMMA. Overnight the company was GONE, and I had to figure it out. I had a tough time at first figuring out what to do. I built an entire vision for my life around this company. Still, to this today have such a VIVID vision of me standing on stage, talking to 10,000 plus people inspiring them to take control of their MIND BODY and SPIRIT. I had built a close relationship with BK, the owner of VEMMA. At this point, right before everything happened, I had lost over 130 pounds. They were about to fly out a full video crew to make a video and more about my body transformation on the products and the company. Overnight everything changed. However, everything I learned in those three years made that pain completely worth it. I had built such a solid base of MINDSET and HABITS that nothing could stop me. I do not regret a thing about those three years with VEMMA. Without that opportunity, I don't know where I would be today. I feel beyond blessed to have met such INCREDIBLE people in those three years.

Now, I have lost over 150 pounds and have had 2 excess skin removal surgeries on my: waist, hips, butt and chest. When you lose that kind of weight, it is pretty standard to have some droopy excess skin. I was blessed with having the resources I have to get these surgeries done. They are not cheap but in my opinion, completely worth it. After my 2 skin surgeries, it felt like honestly a new chapter starting in my life. It gave me such a new level of confidence. Hard to grasp the next step when you see all this droopy skin reminding you of your past. Now at this point, I am 260 with plans of doing a bodybuilding competition next fall. Looking to be around 210-215 with my 6 pack abs and absolutely shredded. The reason I want to do a bodybuilding competition is that I believe it will give me that emotional impact I need to push me to my ultimate goal of 6pack abs. I will be walking across that stage next fall. I will be either embarrassing myself because I didn't put in the work needed to get there or I will be CELEBRATING at the ULTIMATE COMPLETION of my body transformation. From 400+ pound morbidly obese kid to 6pack bodybuilding MAN!

Notes

PART 1
Mindset and Habits

CHAPTER 2
Foundational Mindset

YOUR MIND

Over this next chapter I will be laying down the foundational information needed to understand how: YOU CAN BE HAVE OR DO ANYTHING AND EVERYTHING YOU WANT IN THIS WORLD! Your mindset is truly the FOUNDATION of your results in your life. Your belief system, what you think is real about you and the world around you. Think about this, you are in a terrible car accident and lose most of your memory. Everyone tells you that you are Dwayne Johnson. You need to get back to lifting and making movies. Do you think your life would be different than it is now? Of course, you have a different perspective and set of beliefs on who you are. As you read forward to keep that open mind on the information. Most of the information you will hear is very simple to understand. However, your mind will push you. You will have moments of…. "I am different"….. "this may have worked for you but it won't work for me"…. "I have done this." That's your brain, scared of change. Change is terrifying for the brain. It wants to keep you alive and what keeps you living is to keep doing the same things you are used to doing. There you are safe because you know it. Now, that same thought process has you at this point right now. Still wanting more. Not where you want to be. So remember the definition of insanity is doing the same thing over and over again expecting a different result.

FOUR LAWS TO SUCCESS

I would like to share the four foundational laws to success you must know and UTILIZE to BE, HAVE or DO anything you want. From getting your ideal body. To make the desired amount of money. To have an incredible emotional state. This information came from one of my mentors Kevin Trudeau. He places these 4 foundational principles that will control all the decisions you will ever make. The reason why I am starting with this before anything else is; you will begin to understand as you learn how to implement these four principles in not only your body but the rest of your life.

The first law is: "Who do you listen to?". Another way to state this is, "Who do you take advice from?" or "Who do you allow to INFLUENCE you?". Now we are given advice and opinions each second of every day. How we should eat. How we should sleep. How we should drink. How we should speak. How we should think. What I would HIGHLY recommend you do is to listen to:

1. People who have what you want in that specific area.
2. People who have been where you are at.

For example, over the last 5 years, I have SUSTAINABLY lost over 150 pounds. Let's say a friend comes to me, who is also 400+ pounds and starts asking for advice on how to lose weight. I give him my opinion on BLANK DIET and WORKOUT ROUTINE. He then thanks me and looks at doing that plan also to lose weight. Now one of his friends asks what program he is doing, who is also very overweight and is told what I told him to do. After his buddy says how that will never work or that's bad….. This is an OPINION or INFLUENCE. So take the information in…. ask yourself.. Who should I listen to? Should I listen to David? He has lost over 150 pounds and has been where I am…. orrrrr do I listen to my friend who says that's stupid and won't work but is still fat?? Well, I would hope you listen to me and take my information because I have the RESULTS you are looking for. So, I have information and knowledge the other doesn't.

As you are USING this first law to success, you will notice good people may be giving you contradictory information. We will all run into this situation of SINCERE IGNORANCE. SINCERE IGNORANCE is the idea that your close friends and family SINCERELY wish the best for you; however, they are IGNORANT to the fact they just don't know what they don't know. For the most part, friends and family don't intentionally give you poor information. They just don't know and are doing their best to provide you with good advice. It can be hard to love someone and when they give you advice not to take it but that is something you have to realize. Love and influence are two different things. I believe Tony Robins says it best. Love your friends. Love your family. However, CHOOSE your PEERS. Who is a PEER? A PEER is someone who you are ALLOWING to INFLUENCE your DECISION or EMOTIONS. Now, this does not mean just advice for nutrition and workouts. INFLUENCE is anything that affects your decision making. A great example is a struggle of losing weight in a family or friend group full of overweight people. What will most likely happen during your weight loss journey is friends and family during events will try to get you off of your nutrition and workout routine. Many of us have been there. The uncle who says, "Just one piece of cake won't kill ya" or the mom who says, "Come over for pizza tonight." What happens in these situations is the subconscious ability to try and kick people off their tracks of success because they are worried about two issues:

1. you will be successful in your weight loss, and it will make them feel bad about themselves that they couldn't do it and you did.
2. people become worried that you will leave them because you are changing and they are not.

This pattern is rarely a conscious decision. Meaning, they are not aware of how they are making your life more difficult. They are doing into subconsciously. Meaning, it's an unaware habit they don't think they are doing. So, when this does happen during your body transformation know friends and family don't mean to hold you back. They really do love and wish the best for you but can be doing things that will hold you back from your transformation.

As you look to find mentors take into account that I believe there are six areas to life: physical, mental, spiritual, social, relationships, business. You will not find just one person that fits all of these categories. Take your time to really look at those 6 areas in your life. Which ones do you value most first and which you find the least important. They are all important, but we all appreciate certain things more than others. You can use that positive momentum in growth in one area to pull you forward in others. Once you find which areas you find most important, focus on finding people you can learn from in those areas. My recommendation is you start with: physical, mental, and spiritual. These areas have the most profound changes in our energy and feelings.

The second law is: "TEACHABILITY INDEX."

"The beginning of wisdom is this: Get wisdom. Though it cost all you have, get understanding."
—Proverbs 4:7

TEACHABILITY INDEX

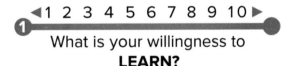

What is your willingness to
LEARN?

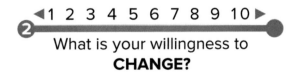

What is your willingness to
CHANGE?

What is the TEACHABILITY INDEX?

1. What is your willingness to LEARN? (rate yourself 1-10)
    a. are you willing to put TIME and MONEY to LEARN the information?

2. What is your willingness to EXCEPT CHANGE? (rate yourself 1-10)

    a. Are you willing to put down what you love most to do for a short amount of time to create the life you truly want?

Multiply these numbers together, and that will give your TEACHABILITY INDEX. What does this mean to you? Many of you reading this book will feel this is not your first book. Or maybe you find yourself trying new things but have a hard time doing the things that people recommend for you to do. You could be willing to spend your last dollar and read this book, but if you are not willing to adopt this information into your everyday life and EXCEPT that CHANGE is involved, you will NEVER CHANGE.

It is a humbling experience as you learn and desire change in your life just how little we all know. That is such a great place to be. Do to the internet and a FLOOOOD of information we have all become so cynical to the knowledge that, WE KNOW IT ALL. Stay teachable my friends :) It is such a great place to be. Just because you went to school and have a degree. The learning is not over. The quote I say often is, "MOST PEOPLE DIE AT 25 BUT DON'T GET BURIED TILL 75." We tend to lose our TEACHABILITY. We all have Neuroplasticity. What is Neuroplasticity? The brain can learn and adapt. Your mind is always adaptable. We create this false sense of IGNORANCE of KNOWLEDGE. Stay a life long student.

> *"Known hells are preferable to strange heavens"*
> —Les Brown.

The brain does not like change. What is the brain made for? It is a simple purpose in life is to keep you alive. It isn't to make you happy. It isn't built to help you get what you want. It is there purely to keep you breathing and reproduce. So when change is brought up, your brain is thinking, "ehhhh I don't know about this."… "I have never done this before." … "If I haven't done this before there is a possibility it could kill me now." … "At least you are alive now."… "Let's stay here"… "It's safe."

How can people keep going back to significant others that treat them terribly? It is because their fear of the unknown is more terrifying than dealing with a known hell. Change is scary. Uncertainty is a part of life but focuses on how the possibility for more and better later can change everything.

The third law is: "TRAINING BALANCE SCALE."

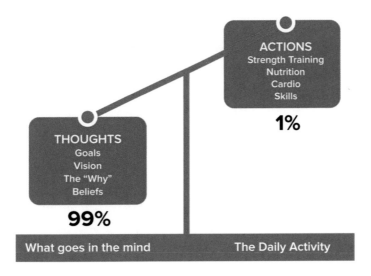

TRAINING BALANCE SCALE

ACTIONS
Strength Training
Nutrition
Cardio
Skills

1%

THOUGHTS
Goals
Vision
The "Why"
Beliefs

99%

What goes in the mind   The Daily Activity

Many people struggle with this. So many people get caught into the struggle of needing to know more. I can't start until I know exactly how the physiology of carbs move into the body so I can make the "right decision." The need to learn HOW to lose weight. Daily, I get messaged on Instagram or asked, HOW DO YOU LOSE WEIGHT?! WHAT DID YOU DO? WHAT'S THE SECRET? Too bad I already know they are missing the most significant point to making a drastic change for whatever poor habit you have. It has almost NOTHING to do with the HOW. HOW TO RUN. HOW TO EAT. HOW TO DRINK. HOW TO LIFT. Your struggle does not come from the lack of knowing HOW. Success in ANYTHING is 99% on WHY it is important to you, and 1% is actually on HOW you do it.

Your THOUGHTS make up 99% of your success. Why do you need to change? What does it mean to you? There is sooo much power in knowing WHY you do something. Just a few days ago I was sitting down with a new friend of mine. I met him through Instagram, and he reached out after we worked out once together because he needed someone to talk to. He was struggling with his body and work. He utilized the KETO diet plan to lose over 100 pounds and was let go from his job. He had started to relapse into old habits eating poorly. So sitting down over dinner we began to talk about life and connect. As I began to give him these 4 basics to success, he began to resist on this area. I asked him, what's more important, the how or the why? He told me, "David, I don't believe in that motivational crap. I got to where I am now purely on the understanding of hard effort and commitment." I looked at him and laughed. I said, "that's great, you have done so freaking well. Are you at your goal? Or are you falling back?". This hit him hard. I could see it was a realization for him. Know that raw determination can get you a very long way but knowing WHY this is important to you will keep you there.

Diving more in-depth into your THOUGHTS.

What goes into your mind….
- Goals
- Vision
- Dreams/Desires
- Imagination
- Motivation
- Beliefs
- Enthusiasm
- The "WHY"
- Standards

Diving more in-depth into ACTIONS…

- The physical activity……
- NUTRITION
- MEAL PLANS
- WORKOUT ROUTINES
- CARDIO
- HIIT
- LIFTING

This is where to transformation REALLY comes from. Where your life TRANSFORMS forever. When your VISION is clear enough. When your BELIEFS change. When your STANDARDS raise. Your life will NEVER be the same. Why? This is where everything changes because when you transform your THOUGHTS, the ACTIONS become ENJOYABLE. When your THOUGHTS are not right, you will EVENTUALLY quit. MOTIVATION or GRIT can only take you so far. People miss it, they focus on the ACTIONS. What nutrition plan? What workout routines? Are these ACTIONS important? OF COURSE, however, you will NEVER sustain those actions for the length of your life if your MIND isn't right. I want to teach you how to TAKE CONTROL of your life FOREVER! Not just give you a nutrition plan and workout routine where you can see success for a short while. I want to teach you the REAL DEEP levels of success in your BODY and your MIND and your SPIRIT.

4 STAGES OF LEARNING

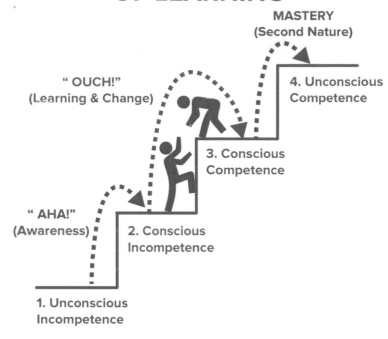

MASTERY
(Second Nature)

4. Unconscious Competence

" OUCH!"
(Learning & Change)

3. Conscious Competence

" AHA!"
(Awareness)

2. Conscious Incompetence

1. Unconscious Incompetence

The 4th law to success is: the 4 stages of LEARNING.

No matter what you are trying to learn. From how to golf to how to be fit. There are 4 levels of learning you will go through. Once you are aware of how to learn and the stages involved, it will help guide you and keep you on track.

The first stage is: UNCONSCIOUS INCOMPETENCE.

Let's break this down. What does UNCONSCIOUS mean? UNCONSCIOUS means you are UNAWARE. So first you are UNAWARE of something. What does INCOMPETENCE mean? INCOMPETENCE means you do not know the information. So put that together. YOU ARE UNAWARE THAT YOU DON'T KNOW THE INFORMATION. This is how most people live their lives. They are COMPLETELY UNAWARE of the amount of KNOWLEDGE there is out there. This is such a

DANGEROUS place to be in life. When you sit at this level, you can NEVER grow. You will live with this idea that I KNOW IT ALL. Which makes you know NOTHING. Now, don't over think these 4 levels of learning. In the end, I will simplify what I mean by all of this.

> *"The only true wisdom is knowing you know nothing."*
> —Socrates

The second stage of learning is: CONSCIOUS INCOMPETENCE.

This is SUUUCH a POWERFUL place to be. When you get to this level of learning the doors open up to a possibility. What does CONSCIOUS INCOMPETENCE mean? Let's break it down. What does CONSCIOUS mean? CONSCIOUS means you are AWARE of it. You see something. What are you AWARE of? You are AWARE that.... What does INCOMPETENCE mean? INCOMPETENCE means, do not know the information. So put them together. YOU ARE AWARE THAT THERE IS INFORMATION AND KNOWLEDGE THAT YOU DON'T KNOW! This is where you bring back your previous STUDENT life in you. This is HOW you become a student once again. Understand there is knowledge that you don't know right now that can help you BECOME the individual you want to be!

I was having a conversation with a guy at the gym. He was probably in his mid-20s. He seemed very confident in knowledge in the gym. However, this guy was about 15-30 pounds overweight with a little belly. You could tell he was not a lazy person. This guy was unaware of my weight loss and knowledge of weight loss. We got in a discussion about the body and what's healthy and how to lose weight. As the conversation started to rise, he had made the statement to me that he knew it all. I knew at this point no matter what I brought to his attention in facts would not impact this person. He had gotten to a place where he believed he knew it all. Whether you are at a point of being completely ignorant to all things fitness or you are at this place where you think you know it all. You are now going to stay where you are. You can only go as far as your mind will allow you to learn new information and use it.

The third stage of learning is: CONSCIOUS COMPETENCE.

Let's first break it down. What does CONSCIOUS mean? CONSCIOUS means that you are AWARE of. You see it. What does COMPETENCE mean? COMPETENCE means you UNDERSTAND THE KNOWLEDGE or INFORMATION. SO YOU ARE NOW AWARE AND KNOW THE INFORMATION. This is where you will spend much of your life. Learning new information from a MENTOR. You will USE this information in your own life. However, you have to really THINK about it.

When you are learning how to squat correctly. You will have some COACH or MENTOR teaching you. Once they TEACH you this NEW INFORMATION what happens? You get there. Step under the bar and THINK….. "Where do my hands go?" Ok, there that's right. As you start your squat, what's going through your head? You have to really THINK about it. "Ok, High chest. Tighten my core. Keep my knees out over my toes. Don't buckle my knees. Get deeper. Push through the heels. All of this information you have to indeed THINK about during the squat to make sure you are doing it right.

The fourth stage of learning is: UNCONSCIOUS COMPETENCE.

Let's keep it simple. Break it down. By this point, you may understand. What is UNCONSCIOUS? It is to be UNAWARE. OR you don't THINK about it. What is COMPETENCE? You KNOW the information. SO YOU ARE UNAWARE THAT YOU KNOW THE INFORMATION. Most successful people got to where they were by UNCONSCIOUS COMPETENCE. There were completely UNAWARE that they were just doing the RIGHT things. Another way you can think of this is AUTOPILOT. You have been thinking about doing something over and over again till a point now that you can do it without putting mental energy towards it.

You have been lifting for a few months now. Your coach has been critiquing your form for months. Squatting over and over again. You get to this point you hold PERFECT form without even thinking about it anymore. You are now UNCONSCIOUSLY COMPETENT on how to squat. Do you remember when you start to walk….. "ok, heel toe heel toe." "Lift foot…. swing leg…" OF COURSE NOT. You went through the failure rounds of learning so young and do it with such a level of AUTO PILOT that you just DO IT without thinking. YOU CAN DO THAT WITH ANYTHING AND EVERYTHING IN YOUR LIFE! You can and will get to a point where eating healthy choices isn't even a thought. Going to the gym takes almost no motivation or effort. This is so because you have created it into a HABIT.

Most of your life is in AUTO-PILOT. You drive certain ways because you always have. You eat certain ways because you always have. You think positively or negatively because you always have. You surround yourself with a particular type of people because you always have. How often do you question your AUTO-PILOT? We are nothing more than patterns you brain uses because it has to. There is way too much going on to think about what you are doing actively. It's all a sequence of patterns you were given or learned at a very young age. So question how these patterns are affecting your life. Are they helping you or hurting you?

These four foundational principles to success will help guide you on your journey to create the best version of YOURSELF. I said, YOURSELF. This is YOUR life. No one else. You have YOUR journey. You may be doing this on your own however you are not alone! Take 100% responsibility for your life. All the mistakes you have made. All the significant decisions and success you have had. There is something POWERFUL knowing that you are in control. So many people have the victim mentality that it's not their fault. It was their parents. It was where you grew up. It is my genetics. There is something SO POWERFUL knowing that you have just been unaware of how to make the RIGHT decisions. That means if you change a few things in your life EVERYTHING changes! (1)

YOUR DRIVING FORCES

THERE IS NO SUCH THING AS AN INNER ENEMY

What's wrong with me?....Why am I such a failure?... I am broken... We all have said that in our lives. Looking for that gremlin that's inside moving strings around to keep you from where you want to be. This is a HUUUUGE realization to come to. You do not have an inner demon controlling you. You are not broken. You can REALLY let go of old beliefs like that. No matter what you are doing. From binge eating to sitting and playing video games all day. You are doing it because some part of you thinks it needs to for being of who you are. Based upon your view of the world and the experiences you have had, you believe deep down these behaviors are necessary. Whether these patterns were created through family history or a traumatic event. We all have habits that hold us back but fill a "necessary void." For example, many people who binge are feeling they have a piece of them missing. Either not truly happy or genuinely feel loved...etc. So their pattern is through eating that fullness works to fill that void.

EVERY BEHAVIOR AND HABIT YOU HAVE HAS A POSITIVE INTENT BEHIND IT

So you have a struggle with binge eating. What you have to realize is your mind has rationalized that habit to fit for positive intent. The feeling of a full stomach in your brain gives you a sense of feeling full emotionally. So when you binge eat, you are filling this "void." Or maybe every time you start a new nutrition plan you quit in the first few days. Perhaps you are noticing how your friends are resenting your decisions to eat healthier and in doing so worried about losing them. So you quit keeping your current friends. No matter how weird or quirky those behaviors may be. You have created some logic in your mind justifying those behaviors. What's also important to know with this poor behavior is that you are doing the best you can with the knowledge you have been given so far. Very rarely do we look at our actions and ask our selves, where did this behavior come from? Is it supporting my life? Is it hindering my growth? Keep these two FOUNDATIONAL UNDERSTANDINGS in your mind throughout this book.

1. THERE IS NO SUCH THING AS AN INNER ENEMY
2. EVERY BEHAVIOR YOU HAVE HAS A POSITIVE INTENT BEHIND IT

The DRIVING force

Within our beliefs, they are shaped to do one of two things. Either the acquiring of pleasure or the deterring of pain. Everything we do comes from this simple understanding that we are attempting to get comfort or avoid pain. This sounds so simple, maybe too simple. Think about it. Are there things you are doing that you know you SHOULD be doing, but you aren't? When you are putting something off what are you doing? Let's say at the gym. You KNOW it is good to go to the gym and workout, but you don't do it. Why is that? You are imagining the PAIN involved to hit the gym. The pain of pushing your body to failure. You don't want to feel that pain, so you procrastinate going to the gym. Let's push that procrastination back even farther. Your body gets even worse. At some point, you get this overwhelming feeling of pain at the moment that if you don't change you will die or be in more pain than the workout. So what do you do? You Workout! You associated more pain with NOT going to the gym than going.

Most people have a belief system that losing something is worse than the possibility of gain. Which of these scenarios creates more of an emotional connection to you?

You sit here reading this book. Taking this information and using it in your life. You have a MASSIVE transformation in your MIND and BODY. Deciding to take MASSIVE action in the gym. You take MASSIVE action changing your NUTRITON to proper NUTRITION. Based upon fueling your body. Instead of eating for pleasure. In a year, you lose 100 pounds. You create the IDEAL shape for yourself. You look at yourself in the mirror so proud of the DECISION you made. Taking 100% responsibility and control over your life. Your energy levels are so much better giving you the ability to do more each day of what you enjoy to do. Your friends and family around you are so proud of you. They celebrate the results you have created.

Or you don't make the decision to take control of your mind and body. You set this book down and think to yourself. "This is only for him. Maybe others will see great results from this book, but I am different. I can't change. I have tried". So you keep making the same decisions you have always made. You eat for pleasure. You sit on the couch and distract yourself, by watching TV and playing video games, so you don't see how poor your body is functioning. Sitting on the couch all day has made you moody and depressed. Friends and family don't want to hang out with you because you are so unhappy. Not only that you have a family. You have three kids, and all of your kids begin down the same road as you. Your kids take the example of the life you have lived as their own. They begin to eat for pleasure and become lazy and moody. They get to school, and kids start to mock them senselessly. They come home each day from school crying their eyes out. Screaming they wish they were never born. All because they followed the habits of you. They have used you as a reference for how to live life, and you FAILED them.

Which one of these situations makes you feel more emotionally attached? I know for myself the idea that my poor habits can be adopted by my kids and they can fall into the same sense of failure has me terrified. That brings me so much emotional connection that I will NEVER allow myself not to live the best life I can because if I don't my kids could fall into the same problems I went through. That PAIN thinking that I could destroy my kids' life is powerful.

It is about understanding how PAIN and PLEASURE control your life and the decisions you make. Recognized how we use the avoidance of PAIN and the acquiring of PLEASURE to dictate our decision making. What we may not see how in the background out of our focus how much PAIN or PLEASURE that action is making in your own life. The little PLEASURE of eating a Snickers bar to feel that sugar rush. Is that worth all the PAIN later on of being fatter and more sluggish than ever before?

I believe that our decision making comes not from even the ACTUAL PAIN or PLEASURE of a situation but our BELIEFS. The certainty of what we think to be true. Specific action will either lead to PLEASURE or PAIN in the future. This means that we are not even making our decisions of the REALITY of the situation but what we BELIEVE is the REALITY.

"If you distressed by anything external, the pain is not due to the thing itself but to your estimation of it; and this you have the power to revoke at any time."
—Marcus Aurelius

What brought me to be so PAINFUL about life at such a young age? At an age where really there is not a lot to be worried about. At the age of 18, I was already 400 pounds. Seeing how destructive that was on my body already. I was on two different meds for Pre Diabetes and blood pressure medications. Countless doctors were telling me what I was going to deal with in the future. I had created this reality of pure PAIN dealing with this problem for the rest of my life. Not only dealing with it but thinking it would NEVER be fixed. I made an estimation in my mind of how much PAIN it would take to get through it not only that I believed that I was too far gone. A point that you can't come back from.

Looking back at the ACTUAL struggles I went through throughout the process of my weight loss up till now, there wasn't a lot of ACTUAL PAIN involved. Was there some? Of course, some times the gym was very tough. I went through: cramps, pulled muscles, lean meal over pizza, water instead of alcohol. However, looking at the PAIN, I estimated it would take to get through it wasn't 10% of what PAIN I ACTUALLY FELT to go through the process of losing over 150 pounds.

Activity

Let's take control of a few actions you have been putting off.

First, let's make a list of 3 actions you have been putting off to take more control over your body. Maybe you need to throw away all the junk food in your house. Or perhaps you have been putting off going to the gym. Or perhaps it's getting a gym membership. Possibly it's getting rid of all the pop in the house. Maybe it's your pattern of binge eating.

After you have your list. Write down the answer to this question next to each action: What pain have you associated with this action that you have not done it yet? Why haven't you taken action? Be honest with yourself. That is one of the hardest things to do. We have all been so good at not being honest with where you are at. So think about what REASONS have you connected to not taking action.

Next, take your list and think about what PLEASURES have you received from doing the action you know you need to change. What PLEASURES have you felt from binge eating? What feelings of PLEASURE have you received from not going to the gym? We all have a desire to get PLEASURE and avoid PAIN. It's all about creating better ways to prevent PAIN and gain PLEASURE, without it causing more pain farther in the future. Being productive with our choices. I know you don't want the feeling of "starving" yourself of what had given you pleasure in the past. Most of these pleasures, as you will see, will be coming from the instant gratification of feelings.

Fourth, write down what it will cost you if you don't change now. This is where we can see how much PAIN you are putting on yourself because you have not to make the decision to change. What will happen if you don't take control of your nutrition? What will it cost you if you keep filling your body with all the crap you have been filling it with? What will happen 3 years from now emotionally? Create that VIVID image of what will it cost you not transforming your body 10 years from now. Don't make it something simple like, "I will be sad" or "I won't be happy." Be as detailed as you can. Who will you hurt? Who will you fail? How will your emotions be? How will your kids see you?

The final step, write down all the PLEASURE that will come from taking ACTION on what you know you need to do RIGHT NOW! Write a POWERFUL list of PLEASURES that will come from taking action TODAY. How will you see yourself in 5 years knowing you took ACTION for 5 years and have succeeded? How much deeper are your relationships? How does your energy feel? How do your friends and family see you after you took control of your body for 5 years? See how your life will be positively affected by taking ACTION today and how it will look years into the future.

Now, set down this book. Take as much time as you need. Do this exercise. The more energy and focus you give it the more real it becomes. We see how PAIN and PLEASURE control our daily decisions. These decisions control our actions. Our actions control our daily habits. Our daily habits control our lives. Take this exercise seriously. It could be the difference from having your IDEAL body and looking back 10 years from now feeling the weight of a thousand tons of stress and regret not making the change in your life. (2)

Habits

You are on the phone with your significant other, in the middle of a deep conversation, you are walking to your car. At that moment the discussion gets more intense. You get into the car and turn it on. Then, remembered you forgot something in the house. So you go inside and grab the item. Come back to the car and then proceed to turn the ignition again, hearing that awful grinding sound. Realizing you had already started the car... Who has been here? I know I have. I literally did that with my mom a few days ago.

So what does that mean? What I am helping you understand is, how much of your life do you really take time to think about and how much are you doing because it's a habit? Day in and day out you are choosing: places to eat, times to wake up, drinks to drink, videos to watch, people to talk to. So much of what we do daily is an AUTOPILOT response. Do you really think deeply about what to have for lunch? How is it affecting your energy? How is it affecting your health? Obviously not because we both at one point got in the habit of eating for taste and convince over fueling our bodies.

The part of life is so dangerous, think about it... How much of your life do you really take time to understand before you make a decision? Or do you just do the thing you did yesterday? Most of our daily habits are entirely subconscious. We do them day in and day out without even recognizing why and how much we do it. Have that speech in a class where your brain melts hearing another one of your classmates say "um" about 2.5 BILLION times. Sitting in a lecture to the person sitting next to you tapping their pencil and not even hearing that they are making a clicking noise. The guy is sitting next to you waiting at the bank who uncontrollably shakes their leg while touching yours.

Becoming aware of your daily habits and routines is so essential to controlling your day and ultimately controlling your life.

How do you control or change a habit? Well first, you have to become aware of how a habit starts. Patterns come from some sort of stimulation. For example, when it comes to the car. Naturally, after you get into a car, what is the first thing you do? Turn it on. So, it's a rare situation that your vehicle is on before you get in. But from time to time the car is on before you get in. The first stimulation are you getting into the car, so naturally, the next routine to the habit is to turn the car on. This time resulting in you to turn on the car after it has been turned on, making you grind the gears.

A more applicable scenario is with eating. I know for me, I created a habit of eating whenever I was bored. So, especially at night, it was a brutal habit.

Whenever I felt bored, my first gut reaction was to go to the pantry to get food. This would give me something to do while I was playing video games watching tv. At this point, I would grab a bunch of chips and pop to be able to inhale while watching tv. The reward would be a full stomach and something to do.

The sequence to any habit is stimulation - routine - reward. Something triggers you to do an action and thus giving you some sort of reward from it.

Boredom eating for me is still a habit that I work to stay away from. The best way to keep yourself from making any bad habit is to stay away from anything that will trigger it or find a new better way to get the reward you desire. So to this day, I work to keep my schedule moving throughout the day and keep myself moving because whenever I sit for long periods, my natural gut reaction is to want to stand up and walk to the kitchen to grab a snack. Thus giving me the reward of doing something.

There are roughly 4 different ways to stimulate yourself into some sort of habit: location, time, emotions, people.

My beach house has always been a haven for me. A place to get away and turn off my phone and all outside stimulation. It is a place to relax and let loose. It is also a place I have been very accustomed to eating my face off with ice cream and pizza. For the longest time, I had such a struggle with sticking to a nutrition plan while at the beach house. Because for the last 20 years of my life, it has been a trigger to eat and let loose. Not to mention that I already had the habit of eating when I was bored. So between not doing much and the location of the cottage, I tended to BINGE EAT while I was there. This habit went on for a few years while I was in the middle of the majority of my weight loss. Never really understanding why I did that at the cottage. Once I became aware of how habits form and are triggered, I worked at keeping myself very focused and mindful not to fall into that trap again. Over the last year, I have gotten much better at not binge eating at the beach house.

Activity

Alright, let's work on 3 negative habits you have. Take a moment and think of 3 patterns you have that you would like to change. Here are some possibilities I have had to deal with in my past: binge eating, eating badly at night, drinking pop, eating sweets, eating poorly at restaurants, eating poorly with certain people, being lazy around certain people.

Make that list of 3 negative habits you have. First, let's find out the trigger. Think back on the last time you made that poor habit. Where were you? Who were you with? What feelings did you feel? Think back to the time before that. Where were you then? Who were you with then? What feelings did you feel then? Have you found any patterns?

When you have seen a design with a bad habit you have, write it down as the trigger.

Now, let's figure out your reward from that bad habit. When that bad habit happens, what do you get from it? Is it satisfaction? Is it a feeling of fullness? Is it something to do? Is it the feeling of fitting in? Is it a feeling of comfort?

Once you have figured out the reward you get from that bad habit, think about other ways you can get that reward. For example, if over time you feel lonely you set the pattern of binge eating. Which the reward for binge eating is feeling full. What other ways can you get the feeling of fullness without binge eating? Maybe it's drinking 18oz of water. Perhaps it's calling a close friend to connect with. Maybe it's watching a heartfelt motivational video. Look at creating a new habit that can give the reward of feeling full.

Once you have all 3 parts down, read it out loud to yourself.

"When I get the feeling of being lonely, I will call my mom for love and support. This will give me the feeling of fullness, for the fact that my mom makes me feel loved and supported."

Everything STARTS with your DREAM.

It's powerful to know that 95% of people NEVER INTENTIONALLY decide what they want. What do they want their body to LOOK like? What do they want their body to FEEL like? What kind of ENERGY do they wish to have? You must start with the VISION in mind. You will have no idea how to accomplish it. How long it will take. Who you will learn from. Before any of that you must create that VISION. At the beginning I aimlessly over and over again tried and failed to transform my body. I started with the HOW. Should I do P90x? OR maybe the Ab lounger. I am going to do KETO. I am getting a gym membership. Just like I explained in the four basics to success, your THOUGHTS hold so much more POWER than the ACTIONS. When your THOUGHTS arn't there, you will eventually quit. I did that over and over again.

Being told HOW to lose weight. However, no one ever told me, WHATS YOUR VISION FOR YOUR BODY? Whats the ULTIMATE VISION for you? The DRASTIC change in my body happened over a little over year timeline when I finally created that SHREDDED VISION. Your IDEAL is not…. "I want to lose SOME weight." Well guess what, you do anything for a day and you will lose SOME weight…. "I want to FEEL better." Well guess what, you wake up the next morning and you will FEEL better…. I want you to CREATE A VIVID DETAILED description of your IDEAL body. Lets figure that out now.

In this activity, we will be diving deep into your IDEAL body. Turn on some music. What does your IDEAL body look like? How much do you weigh? Go online, find what YOUR IDEAL body LOOKS like. Not what you think your parents want. Not what you think the world wants but what do YOU WANT!? Let's go deeper…. How does your body FEEL? How much ENERGY do you have? How much PAIN do you have? How much FLEXIBILITY? How HEALTHY are you? … Let's go even DEEPER….. How does it FEEL WHEN YOU HAVE THIS BODY? How does it FEEL to have the ENERGY you want? How does it FEEL to have the LOOK you want? How does it FEEL knowing you have MADE IT? Below write in the first person, like it has already happened, that you HAVE that IDEAL body.

VISION BOARD

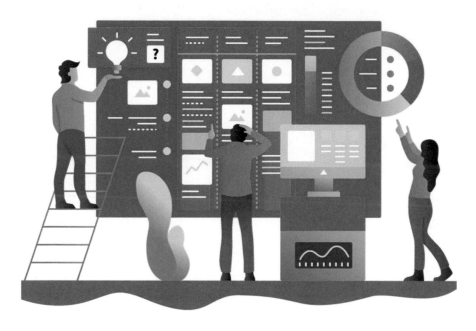

I AM so happy and grateful now that my body is.....

_____

_____

_____

_____

_____

_____

_____

YOU WILL BECOME WHAT YOU THINK
ABOUT MOST OF THE TIME.

How was that activity? Was it challenging to create a vivid picture in your mind? If your first time attempting to make that vivid picture was difficult, you are not alone. Using our IMAGINATION is something we are geniuses at when we are young, but as we get older, we think more "realistic." We rarely allow ourselves to DREAM! To create some ULTIMATE VISION of what is POSSIBLE in our lives. So, what I recommend for you to do is do this activity EVERYDAY for 7 straight days. Creating a more VIVID and IDEAL VISION for your body. I don't even care if you believe you can do it. I just want it to EXCITE you for POSSIBILITY! Once you have a VIVID VISION of your ideal body. I want you to write it down on a notecard. This is your DREAM! Each and every day before your feet hit the floor and heads touch the pillow, you must read your VIVID VISION out loud with ENTHUSIASM LIKE YOU ALREADY HAVE IT! Just envision the possibility of it. I can picture in my head so VIVIDLY….. Me standing on a stage in front of thousands of people in a PINK MAN THONG. Absolutely SHREDDDDED! Speaking to them on the INFINITE POSSIBILITIES you have in your life. I can smell the stage. The oil I put on my WASHBOARD ABS. As I write this, I have an absolute smile on my face thinking of that as a POSSIBILITY in my life. You may not even BELIEVE it yet. That is totally fine! We will get to that later in the book.

We have our SUBCONSCIOUS MIND and our CONSCIOUS MIND. As you read earlier, most people do everything not with CONSCIOUS thought but UNCONSCIOUS DECISIONS. We really don't think too deeply into our daily actions. Do you really evaluate why you are in the job you are in? Do you think too deeply into what foods you eat and why? Do you think deeply about what makes you want to sit on the couch or go for a run? Your SUBCONSCIOUS mind is always taking in information. This is one of the most POWERFUL things that can make it a drastic shift in all areas of your life. Think of your SUBCONSCIOUS MIND as a bucket of water. Nothing is filtering it. Whatever gets put in there stays.

For most of the world, we have terribly dirty SUBCONSCIOUS MINDS. Filled with dirty statements of…. "You are a loser"… "you are lame"… "you are dumb"… "FATTTY"… Filled with the internet telling you that you a victim. You have no control. So on and so on. Now, this bucket is filled FULLL with dirty, awful water. When that water overflows, it's all dirty and mucky. It is too heavy to pick up and flip over. So how do you clean out the bucket? You FLOOOOOOD it with clean, clear water. As you do this, it will slowly become clear and less mucky. As your bucket overflows, it slowly pours out cleaner and cleaner water. Till finally the bucket is cleaned out and all the water inside and flowing out of the bucket is clear fresh water. Your SUBCONSCIOUS MIND is like a magnet. Whatever it is filled with it is attracted to. The water going in is what information you are bringing into your mind, and the water that overflows is the water that is the decisions you make that you are unaware of. So in the past, you have allowed dirty negative stuff to be filling your bucket. All of these negative thoughts and actions of others. With such a dirty bucket you pour out all of these negative actions yourself. So the only way to change this is to POOOOR positive possibility and information into your mind. This action of daily speaking out of your VISION is also known as AUTO-SUGGESTION or an INCANTATION. As you read your VISION for your body over and over again. You express it with ENTHUSIASM your SUBCONSCIOUS MIND will be slowly cleaned out by all of the harmful dark, dirty water that is there now. I have shared my VISION of my IDEAL BODY out loud so often with so much ENTHUSIASM that it has become a piece of me. Those daily ACTIONS have been attracted by how much AUTO-SUGGESTION I give my mind. I say over and over again with ENTHUSIASM the opportunity have to be SHREDDED! Once I created this VISION, it EXCITED me so to figure out HOW to make it happen. This is the big difference between people that will always have a roller coaster in their body and those who keep and sustain it for their life. Is is the VISION of what you want more than HOW to do it.

As you take this VISION and speak it with ENTHUSIASM EVERY DAY, your SUBCONSCIOUS MIND will be filled through the action on AUTO-SUGGESTION. Over and over again you will fill your mind with clean water giving your mind the ability to make clear decisions. Once it is filled your MIND wants to attract more of that into your life. Seeking out the desire to make it happen. Finding people who can help you with your VISION. Seeing different possible workout and nutrition plans that will help you get there. Like attracts like. As evidence by the fact that people with like minds like to be around each other. We all hear the line, MISERY LOVES COMPANY. So when you fill your mind with your VISION, you will naturally be more attracted to making decisions that are like your VISION.

Turning SHOULDS Into MUSTS

How often do you SHOULD all over yourself and others? I should go to the gym. I should eat better. I should not eat that pizza or cookie. This is where most people live so much of their lives. "Shoulding" all over themselves and others. No, how do you go from "shoulding" things to getting them done? They turn into MUSTS. What is a must? A must is only a should with enough REASONS for why it needs to be accomplished.

You have work at 8am. Why do you wake up and get to work? Well, you know that if you don't go to work for a certain amount of days in a row, you will get fired. If you get fired, you can't provide for yourself and others. So pretty much no matter what you make that happen, even if you don't care for your job.

Take this perception into your SHOULDS. I should go to the gym. What will make you feel like you MUST go? Well if I don't go for too many days in a row, I feel sluggish and off. Also, I will start to gain fat. If I gain too much fat I can get certain diseases I don't want to get. Going to the gym for so many consistent days gives you such added energy and focus. Just like the VISION for your IDEAL BODY. You can take those SHOULDS you have and push the worst case scenario out if you don't do it what's the worst thing that could happen? What's the best case scenario if you were to do it every day? Turning SHOULDS into MUST is as simple as making enough empowering REASONS WHY you need to.

CHAPTER 3

Tony Robbins' Triad

This is by far my favorite chapter to write about when it comes to the most incredible transition of my consistent ACTIONS and EMOTIONS. Having the ability to control your STATE is so essential. Most people have no idea where their EMOTIONS come from. Why is it so important to be able to control your EMOTIONS? Well just think about it. When you are SAD, you sit on the couch. Watching a love or emotional movie you have this overwhelming desire for pizza and ice cream. So you take action on this desire and eat your weight in pizza and ice cream to help fill this emotional STATE you are in. Now, just two days later, you are at the gym and frustrated on your poor decisions that night. You are speaking to me and have such an uplifting and inspirational conversations that INSPIRES you to throw away all the junk food in your house and go on a 5-mile walk. This HIGH ENERGY STATE got you to make a significant ACTION of throwing away all the junk food in the house! Most people think it is some uncontrollable river of EMOTIONS that flow them through life. However, that is not true. We have the ABILITY to control and guide our EMOTIONS to create the right ACTIONS in our lives. Your THOUGHTS control your ACTIONS. Your ACTIONS control your RESULTS. Your RESULTS fuel your THOUGHTS to a higher place. So ill ask you again. How awesome will it feel to be able to guide your EMOTIONS to more CONSISTENTLY take the RIGHT ACTIONS to get MORE RESULTS?

People always tell me, "david! You are so happy all the time!", "You are so positive all the time." This isn't because I was born this way. You know from my story I had a past where I was so miserable I almost killed myself. I was able to put on a mask of being happy and having it together, but honestly, in reality, I was a wreck. I can tell you now, from the bottom of my heart that this information brought such a turning point in my life once I consistently used it.

Let me first tell you what this isn't. This isn't some BS mantra of saying… NOTHING IS WRONG, NOTHING IS WRONG, NOTHING IS WRONG. I AM HAPPY I AM HAPP I AM HAPPY. Blinding speaking and sticking your head in the sand in your life to ACT like nothing is wrong. This is the foundation to HOW your EMOTIONAL STATE works. It is also the application of getting REAL with yourself. Getting to the real place that you are in. Not the fake situations we think we are in.

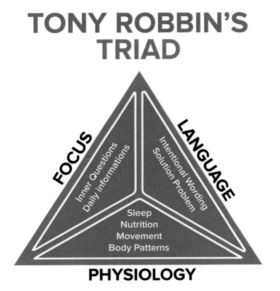

Physiology

Physiology, your physiology is how you use your body. The active movement and placement of your body. Most people understand the relationship between how you FEEL and how you LOOK. For example, If I were to ask you, what does a "sad" person LOOK like? What would you say?….. are they standing or laying down?….. are they spreading out their arms and legs?…. or are they curled into a ball?…. are they breathing deep or shallow?…. are they looking up or down?…. are they smiling or frowning?…. I ask you these questions, and I can almost guarantee everyone reading this book was thinking the EXACT same thing. We mostly realize how our EMOTIONAL

STATE affects or body, but the REAL IMPORTANT understanding is knowing that your BODY AFFECTS your EMOTIONAL STATE.

The ability to raise your EMOTIONAL STATE through your physiology is so important. So when you are sitting on the couch feeling your EMOTIONAL STATE dropping, you can handle those thoughts of wanting pizza to creep up. The desire for ice cream raises. Now, you can stand up. Do some jumping jacks. Just 4-5 and feel how your EMOTIONAL STATE rise and that desire for pizza or ice cream lower. This is why I believe it is so essential to START your day with physical activity. It gets you to a HIGH ENERGY STATE early in the morning. Propelling you through the rest of your day.

Don't just take my word for this. Try it yourself. You will see how amazing it is to feel subtle changes in your emotional state only by tweaking your body. If this isn't your first page of reading. I'm sure you have slowly started to slump in your chair letting your shoulders roll forward. Your head is probably lowering, and your eyes are probably low. You can begin to feel your EMOTIONAL STATE lower. Now in this lower EMOTIONAL STATE, it is harder for the brain to focus intensely on the information. So I challenge you: tighten your core, sit up taller with your chest high, raise your chin and eyes, take a deep breath. Now compare the feeling now to right before you did it. Does it feel different?….. How do you think different?… Did you get a little burst of energy? I did it while writing this, and I can feel my focus jump a bit, and a slight smile just went on my face. I can feel a subtle new burst on energy running through my body.

Focus

Next piece to the triad is your focus. Your focus comes down to the personal questions you ask yourself. We all have that inner dialog. "What am I going to have for breakfast?"…. "Why am I such an idiot?"…. "Why can't a stick to a diet?"…. "Why is this guy so annoying?"… This inner dialog controls our focus and what we see. This is one of the hardest things to change with yourself because you have been asking yourself very similar questions for so long. Remember when I said this wasn't about faking what you are thinking but getting REAL with yourself. To understand that you have to know how your brain really works. At the end of the day, your brain is just a big ol computer. It takes in the tasks it is told and spits out answers. Walk forward.... ok...... stop.... Ok.... smile.... ok. It is nothing more than a computer. So whatever tasks you ask of it, it will do. This is where your inner dialog and focus is so meaningful.

WHATEVER YOU ASK OF YOUR BRAIN IT WILL FIND OR DO. So, when you ask yourself, "Why can't I stick to a diet?" All it knows is...compute.... find old experiences or beliefs that fit the question it is asked. Your brain spits out.... well, your genetics are bad... your family is fat... you are pretty lazy. Do you see the problem with this? When you ask yourself these sorta questions, you will receive answers of EXACTLY WHAT YOU DON'T WANT TO HEAR. Let's unpack it even more too. Does your brain give you EVERYTHING? No, just what you asked of it. So 's comes down to getting REAL with yourself. Most people overestimate the abilities of others and COMPLETELY underestimate their own. Which further pushes you in this false cycle of lack and not enough even though it is not true.

WHY questions are very dangerous. When you ask yourself these WHY questions you are only allowing yourself to see half or less of a situation. "Why can't I stick to a diet?" Then your brain goes out to share with you all of the BS info to gives you a poor self-image. With me, I use to say, "Why don't any girls like me?". This puts my brain into a frenzy finding all bits and pieces of data to fit what I asked of it. Well, David.... you are fat... you are not confident... you don't have abs... you don't have that charisma... you don't have blah blah blah blah blah. You are starting to see the power of what you ask of yourself?

The power of HOW and WHAT questions changes the entire focus of your brain from seeking and destroy to possibility. When you use HOW and

WHAT questions it allows your brain to explore and find hope and opportunity in your mind to grow. "How can I learn to stick to a diet?"… "What can I learn from david that can change how I see myself?"… "How can I learn from my past mistakes to prevent that from happening in the future?" These types of questions allow your brain to work entirely in your favor to execute the task at hand. So when you find yourself asking WHY questions, figure out new ways to change that WHY into a HOW or WHAT question.

To put it into scientific understanding. Your brain is an absolute scientific wonder. It weighs about 3 pounds. There are around 80 BILLION neurons with TRILLIONS of connections or synapses connecting all of these neurons together. In relative terms, if you were to line up all the neurons, with their links in a straight line. It would measure around 10 BILLION meters! That is the distance of going to the moon and back 3 TIMES! That's how astronomical the number of connections in your brain.

Ok, so your brain is crazy complex. Breaking it down one level, that means you have BILLIONS of stimulations happening in the brain every second. The list of physical motions, autonomic systems, thoughts, smells, taste, touch, sight, hearing, feelings. All of these things are simultaneously being transmitted in the brain every second. All this motion in movement and stimulation in your brain there comes to be two step downs before you understand it. After all of this stimulation is happening, you first have your UNCONSCIOUS MIND. The UNCONSCIOUS MIND is roughly capable of processing 11 MILLION pieces of data a second. That means for you that out of the BILLIONS of information going into your brain, your UNCONSCIOUS MIND can only see less than 1% of the stimulation happening.

Diving deeper, there is your CONSCIOUS MIND. The CONSCIOUS MIND is what you actually: see, hear, smell, feel, taste, think. Out of the BILLIONS of stimulation happening in the brain. The UNCONSCIOUS

MIND being able to evaluate around 11 MILLION. The CONSCIOUS MIND, or what you understand, can only focus on about 40 a second. Let that sink in. BILLIONS of things happening all around you every second but you can solely focus on around 40 at a time!

Putting that into terms of your life. Can you create a sense of reality that EVERYTHING is TERRIBLE? Of course, I think your CONSCIOUS MIND can find 40 things or so out of a few BILLION to create the reality you are focusing on.

At the same time, do you think your CONSCIOUS MIND can find 40 things or so that are great things going on? You are right, it can. So when it comes down to it. We are really only seeing such a small piece of the massive amount of things happening to us each and every second.

Why is this important to understand? Going back to my story. You can learn from one of two ways. The successes or mistakes of yourself and others. I have made so many mistakes in my life. The most important, in my mind, is this mistake. My junior and senior year of high school. Billions of things going on, what was I focusing on? Well, let's start with what I had going for me. God blessed me with such an INCREDIBLE support system in my parents. Both my mom and dad would do anything to help me in my life. My father is a Cardiologist making hundreds of thousands of dollars a year. Resources of money was never a struggle. I got my first car before I was even 16 and had my license. I lived in a 7,000 square foot house where we had 5 cleaning ladies clean the house every other week. Changing my sheets and cleaning the entire house. I was one of the most well know kids in all three high schools in our district. I had more friendships than some people will have in their entire life. Every perceived advantage and blessing you could ask for, I had. Now, you would expect, that because of everything I had I was truly happy and fulfilled. We are all given this false doctrine that happiness and joy come from some external situation just out of reach. The new job. The new house. The new body. The new wife. This is so far from the truth. How do I know? I had

EVERYTHING, and twice my junior, senior year of high school. I laid down in my custom shower, crying my eyes out with a pair of scissors in my hands. Cutting at my wrist trying to gain the courage to end my life! How is that possible? With everything right and blessed going on in my world, all I could focus on was what I didn't have. All I focused on was all the PAIN I was in.

Look back at what you just learned about your brain and mind. Even in my reality of so many great blessings around me, are there 40-50 painful things I could focus on compared to the BILLIONS of pleasant things? You can always find 40-50 empowering stuff happening around you. At the same time, you can notice 40-50 PAINFUL things happening around you. This is why FOCUS and what questions you ask yourself is so important. The questions you ask yourself to drive your CONSCIOUS MIND to look through the UNCONSCIOUS MIND and ultimately the BILLIONS of stimulations happening in the brain. I can't undermine how unbelievably important this is for you and your control over your life. (3,4)

Language

Last but not least the final part of the triad is your LANGUAGE. This one is hard especially for the younger crowed reading this book. Younger generations especially have gotten in the habit of using stronger words than necessary to prove a point. You wonder why you people are having a hard time with their EMOTIONAL STATE when everything is either a PROBLEM or ADDICTION. Due to many factors by increasing the intensity of our LANGUAGE we have created more hardship in our heads than need be. The words you use shape the FOCUS you have.

You get into a discussion with a friend, and you disagree with what they are saying. What will cause a more intense response? "I believe you are mistaken" or "You are WRONG." We all know when you tell someone, they are wrong; they begin to get defensive. The language you use with them created a more harsh reply. What sounds worse? Situation or PROBLEM. Think about all the times in your past when things that were nothing more than struggles were first called PROBLEMS. You immediately feel more stressed and anxious about this PROBLEM you have. Now, what happens if that PROBLEM is just a SITUATION or a CHALLENGE. Well CHALLENGES are fun. SITUATIONS can be figured out. PROBLEMS are stressful.

I had a mentor of mine bring this up to me within my own life recently. When I use to tell my weight loss story. I would bring up in my past that I was ADDICTED to food. He, later on, warned me the possibility of creating more struggle with it in the future because I gave it such a hold over me calling it an addiction. As soon as I got in the habit of saying I was fascinated with food. My personal cravings became less desired. Through my language, I was able to make it feel less stressful.

So next time you are talking with yourself or with others be sure you are very active with using the correct language. Your language affects your focus. Your focus affects your emotions. Your emotions influence your decisions. Your decisions affect your results. Be very accurate in your word choice. It may be the difference between a PROBLEM and a SOLUTION.

CHAPTER 4
Who fills your time?

Most of us have been out in the situation when we were young on "momma knows best." Where we start a new friendship with someone. You are having such a fun time with this individual, and your mom comes to you and says you are not allowed to hang out with them anymore. You become frustrated and don't understand but listen to your mother and move on. Years later you see how your friend has fallen off the deep end into a nasty individual and looking back at it you are relieved you did not spend much time with that person. Why is this so important? Who you surround yourself with most is who you become. Most of us have this desire to fit in. So naturally, we will adopt the habits of our peers we are surrounding ourselves with. This pattern keeps us stuck into the same habits that are holding us back from the next level in our lives. For example, remember how I talked about in the chapter on "who do you listen to," I made the example at family gatherings your friends and family will SUBCONSCIOUSLY sabotage your dreams and goals by pushing you to CHEAT. Naturally, because of our desire to fit in, we indulge in these struggles. We tend to make poor decisions around people that make those same poor decisions.

You go out to eat with your same friends and get caught up in this pattern. Your first friend orders the pizza. In your mind…."oooo that sounds good… Followed by your next friend ordering a burger and fries… "oh God, what I would do for a burger right now"… Finally, you are up to order and sitting there with the inner battle marching… "BURGER?"… "Chicken salad?"… "hmm but PIZZZA?!"… "welllll I won't be the only one…. sooooo"… That inner monolog is firing on all cylinders. "Ok, I'll go with the pizza." After this decision is made you are in your head justifying your decision… "Well, you have done great. Having a balance is important. Your friends are eating this way, so it's ok". How many of you have been there starting a new diet? I'm sure all of you have.

You have to remember that who you surround yourself with MOST is who you BECOME. As you make this new chapter in your life to be a better version of yourself, find another group of friends that have succeeded in weight loss or have the ideal body you are looking for. This new friendship will allow you to be pulled up by their new standard of living. You will now be surrounding yourself with people at a different level of habits and decisions pushing you to do the same to fit in.

When I had joined VEMMA. I started to hang around new people. These people had that higher standard set with their bodies. When I would go to dinner with them, they would order meals that fit their nutrition plan. They would talk about proper nutrition and making better decisions. We would have a discussion on books we were reading and what were some of the biggest takeaways we had in our own personal lives. Just like before, I wanted to fit in, so I started embracing these habits also. Pushing me to learn and develop myself. I remember being asked if I wanted to work out with my new friends at the time David and Danielle. They were both considerable fitness enthusiasts. Going to dinner or working out with them was comfortable for two important reasons. They had already made eating healthy a simple part of their lives. Giving me that more natural feeling to make the right nutritional decision at dinner. Also when I would work out with them, they had such joy of the process of working out it made me feel satisfaction from it as well.

Now, this does not mean you get rid of old friends and family. I believe in the 33% rule. In any area of life: Physical, Mental, Spiritual, Social, Relationships, Business. You should spend 33% of your time with people who are better than you. Spend 33% of your time with people at the same level as you. This is important, you should still spend 33% of your time with people that are not at your level. It is crucial to spend some time with others that struggle. Through this time you can help them create new habits and see other possibilities. If you only spend time with people that are better than you or near your level of success, you can never help anyone else in the process.

This will give you such a higher level of growth and desire to hit your goals through the ability to help inspire others.

Some of my most important new RECHARGES for myself once I got really charged up transforming my body was when I would spend time with people in need. Giving them the advice and associations to help them ignite their drive. There is something so motivating knowing through experience that you were an inspiration to someone else. That is why it is so important that you make sure to spend some of your time with people that may not be at the goal body you are looking for. These connections can bring such inspiration to others which in so doing can RECHARGE your desire.

Having a sit-down with someone looking to make a change with their body. You sit there connecting with the individual. Hearing their struggles and poor habits. This opportunity to join with someone that could have been in the same situation as you can give you such great compassion and connection to where you were and how far you have come. Giving you the power to see the road farther ahead as an opportunity, not a struggle.

"As iron sharpens iron, so one person sharpens another."
—Proverbs 20:17

Workout Buddy Traps

One of the most significant warnings I will give someone in this chapter is the WORKOUT BUDDY TRAP! There are two nasty situations I will warn you about that can set you up for failure in the gym. These two decisions will set you up for a good chance of disappointment in the future. What I like about this information is it really came from my own personal experiences. Not from listening to someone else and using it but I seemed to notice how so many people were making these big mistakes.

The first warning is the desire that you need a workout partner. So many people get caught up in the TRAP that you need someone there to MOTIVATE you to the gym. "If I could just find someone that would be my partner. It would be so much easier to go to the gym." I'm sure you have said that a few times to yourself over the years. Looking back at my transformation I realized how many WORKOUT PARTNERS I went through. Going into my final year at CMU, I was swamped. I was taking 19 credit hours of 400-500 level Biology and Chemistry classes with labs. Not to mention building my business in VEMMA. Still finding time to have a social life and workout for 2-3 hours a day. Due to my school schedule, the only time I could make to put in the necessary hours of working out was 5:30am lifts. Now at this point of my journey, my VISION was so clear it EXCITED me every morning and night. So the DECISION was made that 5:30am lifts were going to happen. I was not going to allow myself to let someone else's DECISIONS to hold me back from mine, so I asked no-one but myself to be ACCOUNTABLE for me being there. At this point in time, I had already lost over 80 pounds. Which gave others the thought process that, "If I can be David's workout partner I can be committed to going in the morning." This is such a poor decision on most people. Allowing some outside source to be the source of your choices. Day in and day out. Week in and week out. For an entire year, I held myself to 5:30am workouts. Going through DOZENS of WORKOUT PARTNERS. In my mind. If they showed up, it was great to see. If they didn't show up, it did not affect me. I made the COMMITMENT to MYSELF that I was doing 5:30am workouts. I did not make a commitment to anyone else. This gave me the power to live my life on my terms, no one else's.

Now, if you are new to lifting, it is very important that you use proper form and plan. In this case, you do have a few choices. I would either find a friend to go lift with from time to time to help teach you proper form and a plan. Don't forget from the first chapter to listen to people who have what you want and have been where you are at. Too many people are taking advice from unqualified people. The other option is to hire a personal trainer to teach you the proper techniques and skills in lifting. Personal trainers can be a great asset in helping you try new plans to keep things fun and different while working out. However just like I said earlier. Make sure you think for yourself on finding the right personal trainer for you.

When I made the transition from mostly doing cardio to adding lifting I wanted to make sure I was using proper form. So I hired a trainer to look at my form in lifting. This was such a necessary move. There is a lot involved when it comes to lifting. Much more so than doing basic cardio. Doing squats and deadlifts can ruin your body if not done correctly and at the same time can be huge assets in growing your muscle mass to your ideal body.

The other WORKOUT BUDDY TRAP is thinking it is a smart idea to find someone struggling like you and choosing them to be your WORKOUT BUDDY. So many people make this mistake because they feel that since they struggle with the same thing that they can relate and motivate each other. This couldn't be FARTHER from the reality. Think about it. You are struggling with committing to the gym, so your best course of action is to find someone else having the same struggle as it will help you get through it. What ends up happening is not only do you have to create the motivation for yourself but for your WORKOUT PARTNER too. This makes it such a harder struggle thinking about each day is the person going to be there. You will find yourself not only having to get yourself out of bed but call your partner to do the same. Or laying there in bed thinking, should I call? Are they going? Those types of thoughts only allow yourself more to justify yourself not to go.

Now with that being said. If at this point in time you still would really like a WORKOUT PARTNER. I would recommend to you that you talk to a friend who has already created the pattern of hitting the gym NO MATTER WHAT. Reaching out to him or her and asking if it would be cool to tag along in their workouts. More than likely they will say yes. However, this will still give you the personal power to make decisions on your own accord and not on another. By joining workouts with others, it can help you learn and have fun pushing each other but not allowing the person to control if you go or not. It is YOUR POWER to go to the gym. No one else's.

CHAPTER 5
Beliefs

Beliefs- SEEK or DESTROY

One of the greatest lies we have been told is that events control our lives. Our past experiences and environment shape who we are today. Our past experiences mean absolutely nothing without us placing a belief on what that means to you.

Two brothers were brought up by a single mom. Their mom was significantly overweight. She would eat exceptionally poorly. While they were growing up, they would only drink sugary pop and fast food. Filling their bodies with toxins and unhealthy choices. The mother encouraged them to watch large amounts of TV and video games. They would sit and not often move after school. As these two kids were growing up, they both were also becoming overweight. Getting ridiculed in school, these two boys started having a hard time. As these two kids grew up one became a morbidly obese man. Indulging in the same habits, his mom instilled on him. Not working out, eating poorly. These habits made him feel very poor about himself. Often feeling depressed and anxious about his life.

While the other brother took on an entirely different lifestyle. The other brother ate food to fuel his body. Utilizing proper nutrition and education to fuel his body to live the ideal life. He would eat appropriately portioned meals and drink lots of water. Every day this man would workout to help put on lean muscle and keep himself lean of excess fat. This proper nutrition and workouts brought him lots of energy. Feeling very accomplished and joyous of his lifestyle.

These two brothers were later asked. Why are they the way they are? What you find to be very interesting is they had the same answer. Both men explained how they had such a poor upbringing through their mother. Now where the diverse lifestyle differs later in life is what it meant to them. The obese man says, "Because of my mother I am the way I am, overweight and emotional." The fit man says, "because of my mother I am the way I am. I saw how she lived. I saw how poorly she felt and I wanted to be the exact OPPOSITE."

Now at the end of the day, both brothers had the exact same struggle growing up. However, the difference between the two brothers was what that meant to them. The MEANING they gave that experience. One brother gave the MEANING that I am this way because I will be exactly the same as my mom. The other brother gave the MEANING that will NOT be like my mother. What is the difference? The CHOICE of MEANING you give something.

Believe

What is a belief? Most people walk through their lives thinking with certainty how life is and how they are. Most people believe that a BELIEF is a thing. A tangible object you can look at to prove who you are or what life is. When in reality, all a belief is, is an idea you give certainty to. When you say, you are fat. What you are saying is, "I am certain that I am fat." Now, how did you come to that as an absolute fact?

Through my entire life, until I was about 22 years old, I NEVER read a book cover to cover. Yes, you heard that right. Every class I would either spark note or get the needed answers from youtube or other classmates. I also would do absolutely terrible on writing assignments. I had a BELIEF, from a young age, that I was not a reader or writer. Where did this BELIEF come from? As you would expect, this whole BELIEF, that controlled so much of my life into my early 20s came from a simple situation where I was in slow reading classes when I was in fourth grade. This experience brought me to come to the conclusion that I was just not a reader or writer. How can someone come to that in fourth grade? Why didn't I get better at reading or writing? Well, maybe it had to do with the fact that I would actively go out of my way to read or write because of my false BELIEF. This obviously would make me worse at reading and writing. I rarely did it.

What grade school BELIEFS have you taken with you? That baggage into your mid-20s or 30s or 50s. Look at these BELIEFS as programs in your brain. How do you think your computer would run if you still used the same operating system from high school? Well, that is your brain. You are still using the same programs you made for yourself when you were a kid. Time for an upgrade? I would say so!

Where do beliefs come from?

Let's break down a belief into its more foundational point: an idea. We all have ideas popping in and out of our heads. We don't take too much consideration of ideas. Simple inferences or assumptions to certain things. In doing so, we take these ideas as simple, free-flowing thoughts and do not hold them too close to the heart. What is the difference between an idea and a belief?

Think of an idea as a single building block. By itself, it does not have much control or influence over you. Now when you start to turn that unique idea into a belief, beliefs build certainty into that idea. How do you build certainty into an idea?

A simple metaphor can be used to see how we turn an idea into a belief. Think of your idea as a stool. Your stool becomes stable by how many legs you have attached to it. Your idea has one leg. How stable are you when you sit on it? With one leg you are not very stable. What happens when you put 2, 3, 4 legs on that seat? You become a lot more stable or confident that you will be supported. A leg is a point of reference you have that supports the idea. A reference is some sort of experience you have had in the past that supports the idea. So the more references of past events you place on that idea the more support it gives you.

BUILDING BELIEFS

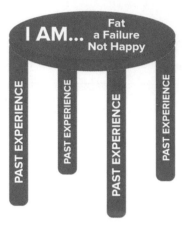

For example, many of you reading this book probably have a belief that you are just a fat person. Well, that belief comes from the idea that you are overweight. With being overweight, you have found examples or experiences that justify or reinforce that idea. What are some reinforcements to that idea? Well, you have probably tried in the past to lose weight and have failed, maybe even multiple times. You probably have been told by friends or family you are fat. Not to mention how many times you personally tell yourself it. You look at your cravings and see how fattening those cravings are. You don't know how to work out. You tell yourself that you don't know how to eat healthily. So now that you have created some references to justify you are a fat person you may think now that's who you are. You have created many past references further creating certainty or belief that this is just who you are.

How do you change a destructive belief?

This will come up over and over again. Throughout this book, I have mentioned the idea of TRULY being honest with yourself. Becoming truthful to yourself is so important, you expect others to be truthful to you but, how true and real are you to yourself?

Let's break down this IDEA that you are just a fat person. This IDEA that has been reinforced with past thoughts and experiences building it into the BELIEF that you are just a fat person. Let's ask ourselves questions. Going back to Tony Robbins's Triad. Questions control our focus. Have you ALWAYS been fat? Well, when I was a child, I wasn't fat. So there was a point in time that you weren't? Yes. How many times have you attempted to lose weight? Once, twice, three times? Have you tried EVERYTHING? Obviously not because there are people that have been in your exact shoes that have made it happen. So there must be just something missing that you haven't done. Are there healthy foods that you do enjoy eating? Of course! Who doesn't like grilled chicken or fish? There are healthier options you could be eating more consistently, right? When you have worked out in the past. How did you feel after working out? Did you feel good? It was an enjoyable action after. Are there others who have been successful in weight loss willing to help you? Well, duh! You are reading this. Not to mention the THOUSANDS of others online that would love to help. Do you know its better to drink water or sugary pop? Yes, smile and laugh at yourself. You know you should be drinking more water and less soda.

How strongly do you feel on your BELIEF now? This IDEA that you are just a fat person. How are those references holding you up? Is it really TRUE about most of your references are obviously not true. These references we have given ourselves to hold up this IDEA that we are fat. They are either not true, or there are a thousand other references you can use to take away those things.

"Man often becomes what he believes himself to be.
If I keep on saying to myself that I cannot do a certain
thing, it is possible that I may end by really becoming
incapable of doing it. On the contrary, if I shall have the
belief that I can do it, I shall surely acquire the capacity to
do it, even if I may not have it at the beginning."
—Mahatma Gandhi

Activity

Now, let's DESTROY some of those destructive beliefs and change them into POWERFUL useful ones. Before you start, STAND UP! Put some high energy music on! RAISE YOUR PHYSIOLOGY! Raise that heart rate. I hope you are reading this in a coffee shop. Make a scene. Think, this activity could be the one thing that TRANSFORMS your body forever! This one simple activity could be the point where your DECISION is made, and you are NEVER the same again.

(Split the page in half one side Destructive Belief another side Constructive belief)

1. Draw out your Destructive Belief.
2. Write those references on those legs.
3. Make an X through those references and write next to them why they are wrong.
4. Once all of the legs are crossed out. Go onto the Constructive Belief side of the paper and write down a new Constructive Belief.
5. Take that new Idea, and let's turn it into a BELIEF. Write down as many references to turn that IDEA into a STRONG BELIEF. (Remember the more references you place on an IDEA, the STRONGER the BELIEF)

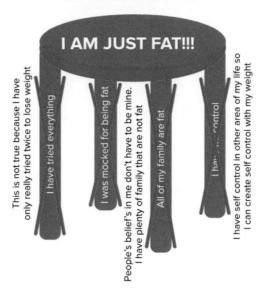

DESTROYING BELIEFS

I AM JUST FAT!!!

This is not true because I have only really tried twice to lose weight

I have tried everything

I was mocked for being fat

People's belief's in me don't have to be mine. I have plenty of family that are not fat

All of my family are fat

I have control

I have self control in other area of my life so I can create self control with my weight

** If you want a more in-depth explanation on beliefs, I would recommend reading the book by Tony Robbins, Awaken The Giant Within.

Accurate Thoughts

This point, one of the golden threads, placed upon the entire first half of this book. However, still, one of the toughest aspects to nail down for the reason that humans tend to reject what they don't understand. It is not something most of you have placed any time measuring or questioning. Accurate thoughts are not something we are taught to work on from a young age, so it is something we don't recognize as a pivotal perspective in our lives.

The first step in working on accurate thoughts is to understand there is a difference between FACTS and INFORMATION. Contrary to popular belief, all the information on the internet about nutrition are not FACTS. Actually, most information on the internet about diet and weight loss is merely people's opinions based on personal experience and not FACT.

I will go into further detail in later chapters on nutrition, but it has almost become a culture fact that fasting is harmful to you. It is "starving" the body. The idea that the most healthy way to live is to eat 3-5 small meals throughout the day. This information does not come to lots of verifiable FACTS based upon no biased research, or for that matter basic logic. Think about it. Up until about one hundred years ago, it was pretty reasonable to have times of feast and times of famine. Where we scavenged and hunted. Our bodies, just like all mammals, can store energy as fat on the body. This fat is there to be used later, in the need that you can't find nutrition to power the body. So this information that states fasting is wrong for you makes absolutely no sense. Especially for individuals with large amounts of fat on their bodies. What is fat but stored energy?

When you question the INFORMATION and look into FACTS, you will see there is very little evidence on "starvation mode." So how has that become such a broad spread idea? It comes from people not questioning INFORMATION and locates real FACTS aka, tests and science to prove. As you read this now, I am on day 4 of a 5 day fast. My energy levels have gone up each day. My focus has gotten better and my cardio in the morning has been better each day.

What this comes down to, within the difference between INFORMATION and FACTS, is the EVIDENCE attached. The reason I have been able to sustain my weight loss for over 5 years is that I have been driven to find the truth, not just information. Looking to see how not only the info sounds but how the evidence proves or disproves it. This principle goes back to the first law of success. Does the individual have what you want? Does the information have sound evidence proving it to be a fact?

This sounds overboard, doesn't it? I have to question everything? My goal and intention of this book are to make you entirely self-sufficient. As Tony Robbins says, "I am not your guru." I am here to share with you how you can do this for yourself. The way I know this works and is sustainable is because

I have been doing it for five-plus years. Focused on control of my mind and body. Isn't this what you want? You want to get over your struggle. These principles will give you the personal power to often make the correct decisions for yourself because you base it on evidence and truth. (9)

CHAPTER 6
Set the Game to Win

As you make this change in your life. You MUST have the mindset this is a LIFELONG decision. This is not meant to be a crash diet course to lose 100+ pounds in 6 months and watch you go back to where you were and worse a year from now. As cliche of a statement, this is: "this is a marathon and not a sprint." Now with that being said. There is nothing wrong with a sprint as long as you have a plan to sustain yourself for an extended period after the sprint is over.

Some people will find much more growth by an all-out sprint to get you in a great momentum. Others will want to start with a couple small decisions to get you moving in the right direction. Either way, as long as the LIFELONG decision has been made, each method is either right or wrong depending on you.

So as you are setting this game to win. Know who you are, know what will excite you and keep you on track. There are a few basics no matter which route you decide to take will keep you on track. This is YOUR life you hold the keys, and you set the rules. So set the standards to make yourself win.

Goals

As I have stated many times before and I will say over and over again. What you think about most of the time is who you become. Goals, dreams, expectations: this becomes your daily game. You will now on, for the rest of your life, become an ACHIEVER. When you write something down and focus on it daily, you WILL accomplish it. Why don't most people achieve their new year's resolutions? Well, there are multiple reasons; however one of the most significant ones that are widespread is no one writes them down and focuses on them daily. As I write this paragraph on my computer, over my right shoulder is my whiteboard, split into three columns. These columns are divided into today, week (....), Month (Oct.). Every day I write on my board what I will accomplish today. On Sundays, I write down my goals for the week and at the end of each month, I write down what I want to achieve that month.

People who continually progress and hit goals keep those goals in front of them. Reviewing them often. Seeing if they are on track. Are they on track to hit it? Do they need to adjust effort or timeline? Be stubborn on your GOALS but flexible on your methods.

Be SMART with your GOALS

Most people don't understand the basics of creating a real goal. A great way to recognize an effective strategy for making a goal is to be SMART.

Specific- Make your goal very specific. Your goal is not to lose weight. It is to lose 45 pounds. It is to lose 10% body fat. By being specific, you allow yourself to be able to track your growth. Tracking progress is ultimately what makes the goal happen.

Measurable- By making it quantitative you can see how progress on your goal is going. This is very important as we have learned you may have to: PLAN, DO, CHECK, ADJUST. The PLAN may change but the GOAL never will. This is why I had spoken about before why your THOUGHTS are so much more important than the ACTIONS.

Attainable- This is where you do have to have some honesty of what body type you are. There is a level of personal love you must have when it comes to your body. You do have a certain level of physiological differences between others. I hate to burst your bubble but many of your most iconic body builders you look up to may take steroids or other PEDs. There is nothing inherently wrong with that but know that certain body types may not be attainable without surgery or steroids.

Relevant - Relevant, this seems out of place but when you think about it. How often do you create a dream or goal that isn't actually relevant to what you truly want? Keeping the outcome and intent is so important. For example, if your ultimate goal is a specific look, make sure that calculated weight is relevant to an actual look you want. The number on the scale helps gauge you, but the goal is a look and feeling.

Timely- It is crucial to creating timelines for your weight loss goals. It is a matter of excitement. Gives you a sense of urgency to hit your target. Creates visions of possibility not too far into the future being at your goal body. Timelines can give you opportunities to look back and reflect on your progress. If you do happen to come up short on your schedule for your goal. Seek out the cause. Was it an effort issue? Do you need to adjust your plan? Do you just need more time?

Keep your Goals in the Palm of Your Hand.

Looking back at an activity you did early on. You had created a dream vision for your IDEAL body. That vision for your body. Full of your emotions, your energy levels, the aesthetic look for your body. You wrote it in the first person like you already had it. I am so happy and grateful now that I am…. Take that statement. That vision for your IDEAL BODY. Write it on one side of a 3 by 5 notecard. On the other side, write down the SMART goals you have down. Each day I do the exact same thing. I read my card front and back before my feet touch the floor and the last thing I read before my head hits the pillow. This primes my head to keep track of my goals and visions for my life. You may make a mistake from time to time. This will help keep those correct decisions in front of your mind for most of the day. If you REALLY want it, I would get laminate covers and keep that card on you at all times.

I can't tell you the countless times that voice was chirping in my ear to eat something NAUGHTY! Driving past Taco Bell, oh my gosh a number 6 combo with a crunch wrap supreme sounds UNREAL right now. Then that immediate decision would turn to me reaching into my pocket and pulling out my card. The front having my VISION and the back side having my GOALS. I would read it giving me that push needed to keep me on track. What you think about most of the time is who you become.

Win the Morning

The power of momentum is so real. This is why having an intentional mourning routine is so so so important. Taking control of your mornings will push into the afternoon and night. As you make the right decisions in the morning, the rest of the day seems so much easier. Success in anything is not BIG decisions of which college to go to or which nutrition plan to choose. It is the almost overlooked benign decisions. Simple choices that compound to make drastic longterm differences. Do I wake up an hour early to get my workout in? Do I wake up little early to read or to watch a motivational video? Do I drink water over a pop?

My mourning routine consists of:
- Alarm- No snooze button
- Prayer and Vision/Goal card
- A tall glass of cold water (12-14oz)
- Youtube Motivational video (2-10min)
- Workout Lift (45min-hour and 15min)
- Cardio (20-30min)
- Read (20-30min)
- Meditation (10-20min)
- Total: 3 hours

Having an empowering mourning routine will prime your day to make it the most affective day possible. I also do intermittent fasting, so my first meal isn't until noon to 2pm. I don't do breakfast. Depending on your work or other obligations you may not be able to do all of these in the morning but the more you can do to start your day off right the better you will be throughout the day. An intentional morning routine will prime your engine for the rest of the day. We all have morning routines or rituals. To most of us, it is an entirely unintentional event. Waking up after 3 to 4 snoozes. Pushing yourself to play catch up. Rushing your shower and any early morning conversations. Acting already like you are just a breeze in the wind with no control. If in your morning you feel so helpless, how do you think the rest of your day will go?

As many of you know, I am a huge fan of Dwayne Johnson aka The Rock. I came up with my morning routine within his morning ritual. I, as many of you, use to say that I was not a morning person. Back in my freshman year of college, I didn't schedule a class till at least after noon. Normally I wouldn't wake up till around 11:30am to noon! Telling myself for years that I wasn't a morning person. I used The Rock as my reference among a few others to take intention in your morning. Pushing off your morning only makes you want to push off all the rest of the things you know you SHOULD do.

Break down the morning routine to hit all the major areas of yourself: physical, mental, spiritual. A portion of your morning routines needs to involved physical activity to prime your body. Get that blood flowing. Followed by priming your mental strength. Reading a book or listening to an audio to help prime your mind.

Last but not least priming your spirit. Whether that is praying to God or thanking the Universe for the countless blessing you have been given is so essential. Priming your soul in gratitude helps keep your stress low and your mind clear to make great decisions.

MORNING ROUTINE CHEAT SHEET

Wake up:

SPIRITUAL:
Bible_____mins.
Pray_____mins.
Gratefulness_____mins.
"_____"_____mins.

MENTAL:
Read_____mins.
Listen_____mins.
Meditation_____mins.
Affirmations_____mins.
"_____"_____mins.

PHYSICAL:
Gym_____mins.
House Workout_____mins.
Walk/Run_____mins.
"_____"_____mins.

RELATIONSHIP:
Good morning txts/calls_____mins.
Gratefulness txt or calls_____mins.
"_____"_____mins.

Total morning routine_____

The Freedom of Discipline

So many people have this misconception of the word DISCIPLINE. This word has been more commonly associated with PUNISHMENT than FREEDOM. We have to DISCIPLINE our children, aka PUNISH them with a timeout or some other negative repercussion. So you wonder why so many people have such a negative connotation to SELF-DISCIPLINE.

Where is an area of freedom most people would like to have? How about time-freedom. The ability to have control over your day. What happens to most people when it comes to their affective use of their time? Well, the average American has the tv on for 3 hours a day. How much time are you wasting each day to things that don't deserve that amount of time? You will be absolutely blown away by how much more time-freedom you have each day by scheduling out each activity. At the end of the night having a few hours to myself to watch a movie or tv show is a gift I give myself for being so disciplined with my time throughout the day. You give yourself a gift instead of regret. There is a huge difference. Creating a schedule to stick to, gives me the comfort knowing at the end of the day I REWARD myself with a movie or show. How do you usually feel after you watch a few shows and see your schedule? Worried and frustrated on how much you need to get done. When you schedule out your day and have the DISCIPLINE to stick to it. You allow yourself to have pleasures that generally would create stress and frustration later by regretting to get things you need to get done instead of a gift you give yourself for a great productive day.

There is something you are striving for. Something that will make your life better. Now, we all know that SOMETHING doesn't come from NOTHING. Consistent ACTIONS must be taken for this to happen. Disciplining yourself to do the countless daily actions that will help guide your life to your ULTIMATE GOAL.

Discipline is the root, the foundation of all the DESIRED results in your life. You can't have ANYTHING without the DISCIPLINE to say YES or NO to the things that will either take you CLOSER or FARTHER from your goal. Not giving in to the SHORT-TERM gratification that will ROB you of your FUTURE DREAM.

Will Smith has become a great teacher on Discipline. "Discipline, that you FORGOE IMMEDIATE PLEASURE for the exchange of LONG-TERM SELF-RESPECT" - Will Smith. Will goes on to explain how he believes that

SELF DISCIPLINE is the definition of SELF LOVE. When you say, you genuinely LOVE YOURSELF. You will do things that a truly LOVING. That means your BEHAVIOR and ACTIONS you take towards yourself are LOVING. So if you are doing things that are hurting your body or your mind, you are not TRULY LOVING YOURSELF. This concept hit me so hard. WHEN you TRULY LOVE YOURSELF, you WILL do the things that will HELP you not HURT you.

> *"The pain of self-discipline will never be as great as the pain of regret."*
> —Anonymous

Power of Chunking

What is chunking? Chunking is the ability to take a huge goal or opportunity and break it down to bite size pieces that you can see and believe yourself to be able to handle. One of the biggest pains was looking at my 400 pound self in the mirror and looking at how I had to lose 200 pounds. How in the world am I going to lose 200 pounds?! Well crazy enough when you chunk it down it doesn't seem so overbearing. Well if you want to lose 200 pounds, can you see yourself losing 2-3 pounds a week? That sounds doable, right? No matter how poor your ability to see yourself at your goal, can you see yourself losing 2-3 pounds a week? Great! You can see yourself chunking that down into the simple idea of losing 2-3 pounds a week. Well, how many weeks do you need to do that for? At 2 pounds a week, in only 100 weeks, you will be at your goal body losing 200 pounds. Doesn't seem so overwhelming now does it? Just drop 2 pounds a week for 100 weeks, and you lose 200 pounds!

One of the most inspirational stories based around the power of chunking is with World War 2 American Army Medic, Desmond T. Doss. If you have ever seen the movie Hacksaw Ridge, it is based upon the true story of one of the most incredible men ever to live. Desmond won the Congressional Medal of Honor, at the Battle of Okinawa.

The quick back story on Desmond is that he was a conscious objector in the war. This meant he didn't believe in carrying a gun or killing anyone during the war. However, he thought it was his duty to serve in the war. Desmond was brought up with a strict view of the Bible. Believing directly never to break the 10 commandments. He was determined never to take a life, no matter the circumstances. Desmond was almost put in jail for his beliefs because he wouldn't hold or shoot a gun, disobeying direct orders of his superiors. With only one option in his mind, the best place for him to be in the war was a medic. Saving lives instead of taking them.

Many of his fellow soldiers did not trust him and out right bullied him for his views. They thought of him as a weakling, and in a tough situation, you could not rely on Desmond. No matter how much he was mistreated he treated everyone with the golden rule. He lived the golden rule, "...do to others what you would have them do to you..." (Matthew 7:12 NIV).

In May 1945, Desmond and other troops climbed the last fortified area on Okinawa. The Maeda Escarpment was a steep cliffside that was the last remaining barrier for the Japanese forces. After the company had secured the top of the cliff, the Americans were stunned when suddenly enemy forces rushed them in a vicious counterattack. Officers ordered an immediate retreat. Soldiers rushed to climb back down the steep cliff. All the soldiers except one.

Less than one-third of the men made it back down. The rest lay wounded, scattered across enemy soil—abandoned and left for dead if they weren't already. One lone soldier disobeyed orders and charged back into the firefight to rescue as many of his men as he could before he either collapsed or died trying.

Everyone left on the top of the cliff was either dead or wounded. Desmond took it upon himself, in the cover of darkness to save as many lives as he could. He pulled at least 75 wounded soldiers out to the cliff side, dead weight lowering their limp bodies down the cliff by a rope. Over and over again, throughout the night he would drag a wounded soldier back and slowly lower them down to safety. Just trying to wrap your head around the idea of dead weight lowering 75 men down a cliff is truly impossible. I am 6'1, 250 pounds. Thinking about myself doing that seems undoubtedly impossible. His quote breaks down the simplicity and power in focusing on simple tasks.

"One more Lord, help me get one more"
—Cpl Desmond Doss.

That quote gives me chills each time I read it. If you were to tell Desmond, you are going to dead weight carry 75 men down a cliffside. What do you think he would have said? That is not possible. The power of focus chunking your goal is so powerful. "One more Lord, help me get one more."…."5 more pounds Lord, help me lose just 5 more."

Day in and day out. Week in and week out. Month in and month out. Year in and year out. Focus on the next logical step of your goal. Chunk that, what seems to be maybe even an impossible goal, down to simple focuses that you know you can hit. Losing 200 pounds may seem too much a leap but how does losing 3 pounds this week sound?

CELEBRATE

You wonder why so many people burn out. You tell me, you grind day in and day out. Restricting your nutrition, working your butt off, for weeks or months and never looking up. What happens to so many people? They burn themselves out. Especially when you get to the more "sustain" stage of your transformation. This may come to a surprise to you, but even when you get to your IDEAL BODY, you can't just go back to eating BS all day and not working out. Haha, that may be a shock to you, but your life will NEVER be the same. You made the DECISION to transform and sustain the new body, that means things will always be different.

I was on Instagram a few weeks ago and read an Insta Story post of a friend of mine, asking how she can stick to her diet. She will do good for a week or two and then totally fall off and binge back. Now, this girl is at a great place with her body, but after talking to her, she wants to sustain it and is having trouble. Well, let's see how you would do. You are eating a very restricted meal over meal. Hitting the gym day after day with no real changes or anything to look forward to. How do you think you would hold up? I would have one heck of time mentally, to keep eating so clean with nothing to look forward to. So what happens? You fall entirely off the deep end not just on one meal but 3,4, 5 days straight of letting yourself go.

This is why finding points to celebrate so vital for the sustainability of your goals. Remember, your life is a marathon, not a sprint. We all know the power of positive reinforcement. Being able to give yourself presents for a job well done. Different gifts give yourself that serotonin boost making you feel good. My recommendation to her was to have 2 unremorseful celebration meals a week. Where you give yourself a no holds bar celebration meal eating whatever you want, no restrictions. Think about it, you eat 3-4 meals a day. Multiply that by 7 days and that's 21-28 meals a week. Being on point for 26/28 meals a week going to really affect your progress that much? It will very little but the mental boost and gratification of gifting yourself those 2 meals. Gives you such an enormous morale boost to keep going, celebrating your good week.

Looking back into college, myself and my roommate Stav, use to have the most EPIC celebration meal habit. After a great week of working out and eating healthy, myself and my roommate Stav use to hit up the local Indian restaurant lunch buffet. I would literally eat my weight in buttered chicken, rice and naan. The smile on my face each week, walking through those doors and sitting down to an unremorseful celebration meal felt so freaking good. We are not talking a little "cheat meal." I'm talking about a solid 3 plater meal, haha. I would stuff my face till my body hurt. The feeling of accomplishment gifting myself this meal was so important. That's why personally I don't like calling them "cheat meals." It may give you the feeling you are doing something wrong. You are doing nothing wrong. You are CELEBRATING a great week of great decisions. Never regret the little gifts you give yourself.

Celebrate your weekly and monthly accomplishments. It doesn't have to be food related. Whatever you feel great gifting yourself for a great job. Maybe it is at 50 pounds down, you go on a cruise. Give yourself future accomplishments, based on results, points to celebrate how well you have done. By celebrating throughout the process, it may be the difference between falling off and sticking through for the rest of your life, never truly falling apart and living in that IDEAL BODY.

Notes

_____

_____

_____

_____

_____

_____

_____

_____

_____

_____

_____

_____

_____

_____

_____

_____

Part 2
Nutrition

CHAPTER 7
Foundational Nutrition

As you can tell, the foundational mindset and habits are so much more important than nutrition. Over half of this book has been hammering foundational mindset and habits because as we move into a proper understanding of food. If you don't feel like you have the correct beliefs or knowledge of habits, you will not stick to any of these nutrition strategies. This is your opportunity, not feeling like you have a grasp of belief or understanding how simple it is to transform your body? Go back to the beginning of the book and reread. Go back through the activities. Break down some of your destructive beliefs and recreate your empowering beliefs. Strengthen that vision of your ideal body. Create more empowering reasons why it is important to take control.

Now, if you are still reading on, the first thing we have to understand is the FOUNDATIONAL knowledge needed to utilize and understand for the rest of your life to always have full control over your body. This information needs to be at the forefront of your mind no matter what nutritional plan you decide to utilize.

When I was talking to my good friend Luke, we were talking about what I should write about in my first book. One of the most unique factors of my story is the vast knowledge and experience I have on different nutrition plans. During my weight loss journey, up to now, I have successfully used: KETO, low-carb, extended fasting, intermittent fasting, carb cycling, macro counting, calorie counting. I can not only tell you about my experience of them but I have done extensive research on each and how the different plans have their foundation in science and why they work. With my Bio Med background and personal experience, I have been fascinated with finding the truth. It's not BRO-SCIENCE but scientific and logical foundation that has brought me to where I am today. Some of it is based in logic, and other is found in actual clinical studies.

Before we get into any specific plan. All plans, no matter what, have a set of foundational understanding of the body. For example, no matter how low your carb intake is if you eat 10,000 calories a day. You are not losing weight. So this information is to help you understand foundational how your body works.

I find nutrition and how the body works fascinating. I know for some of you, just like how a car works, want only the FACTS. I will do my best to carve basic simple facts of, "do this." Mixed with some more in-depth knowledge so you can see the big picture of how it all fits. Like I had said, its not BRO-SCIENCE. So I am going through very in-depth studies that give outcomes, but it's still the human body. There are a lot of things we have no idea how they work together. For example, studies up to now, have said how bad red meat is for you. Out of the newest studies the blame looks to be moving towards the "processed" red meat compared to "non-processed" red meat. (5, 6)

There is only one real aspect of choosing a nutrition plan for you, and that is: it is not about the program as much as how you can stick to it. True longterm success, as we have talked about, is the consistency over time. You have to be diligent in knowing that you have to change your perception of food 90% of the time. Choosing to eat to nourish your body over taste and convenience. 90% of the time, those "CELEBRATION MEALS'" are so crucial for long-term sustainable change. Give yourself times to celebrate how far you have come by eating an entire pie haha. I don't care what that meals are, it won't affect you negatively on the short term, but it will help you mentally for the long run.

Ever been in a class that you are THRIVING in? Out of the assignments in the course, you have all A's. Here comes the final. However, compared to all of your classmates, you don't have to sweat the final. You calculate it out and only need to get a 27% to get an A. While some of your classmates have been putting less than there best and are floating at a C in the class. They are freaking out knowing that to get a B in the course they need to get a 97% or HIGHER. So while your classmates STRESS out, you are watching Game of Thrones because your grade is pretty much locked in.

I want you to take that same perspective in how you eat. Say you have 21 assignments in a class. You ACE the first 19. I am allowing you to be able to FAIL the last 2 and STILL get an A.

Now you have the other class where you do "ALRIGHT." Out of 21 assignments, it goes something like this: A, B, B, D, C, B, C, F, A, B, A, B, C, D, E, D, A, A, A, B, D. What do you get in the class? B or maybe a C? Freaking out along the way on how you do on the Final.

Or you can live life like me. A, A, A, A, A, A, A, F, A, A, A, A, A, A, A, A, A, A, A, F, A. Now what do you get in the class? An A ALLL DAY. What about those two F's? Those two F's were during Game of Thrones time. Because I am doing so well in the class, I can relax and SKIP those two assignments to watch Game of Thrones and CELEBRATE how well I am doing. But because of my consistency of holding myself to a HIGH STANDARD on the other 19 assignments, it is easy to CELEBRATE and ALLOW myself to relax for 2 of them.

The issue is MOST people do "ALRIGHT" on their nutrition, but in reality, they are holding to a B-C average and are pretty STRESSED throughout the semester. When you keep to PERFECT on 19, you can genuinely CELEBRATE the other two meals and still get an A in the class.

Calories

The TABOO word no one likes to hear. What are calories? Calories come down to the amount of ENERGY stored in food. To understand the importance of calories, you must realize what body fat is in its most simple understanding. All body fat is, is stored energy. As you eat calories, if you intake more calories in a day than you burn in activity, you will save that excess energy as stored fat. This stored body fat is intended to be used on a later day. People have to remember, up until about 100 years ago, it was normal to go a few days without eating. Looking for your next kill or finding new edible plants. So when the body is in a caloric surplus, you are often feasting, it takes advantage of that opportunity and stores the excess calories as body fat. Knowing it is most likely to have a famine, lack of calories, being eaten later. So its natural pattern is to save that excess energy.

So the first thing you need to check is what is the IDEAL amount of calories for you to eat a day. What I would recommend is to go on to the internet and google TDEE calculator. You don't need to calculate it yourself. Use the program to see how many calories, on average, to sustain and lose weight. These programs are on average. Which means for the sake of making sure you lose weight, lean on the side of lower calorie intake than higher. Your calorie intake, depending on your: age, height, and weight should sit somewhere between 1500-2700 calories a day. To keep track I highly recommend getting a food tracking app such as MyFitnessPal, Lose It and Lifesum,

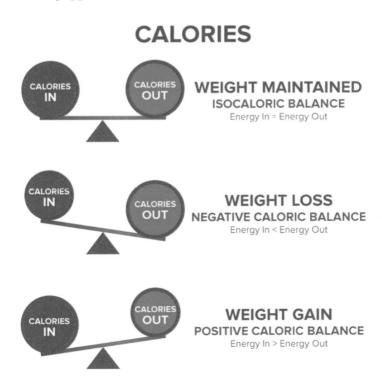

Macro Nutrients

The next step after understanding calories is to understand what Macro Nutrients are aka. macros. Macros are the building blocks for the body and are utilized in different uses. There are 3 macros: protein, carbohydrates, fat. Not all macros are treated equally when it comes to calories. A gram of protein or carbs is equal to 4 calories. However fat has 9 calories per gram. So first understanding how fats can get away from you as you eat is important. It is over twice as dense in calories.

Protein has many uses in the body, but as most people know how important it is for the formation of lean muscle on the body. Protein is broken down into Amino Acids that are used for many functions in growing the body. Your intake of protein should sit somewhere between .5-1.5 grams per IDEAL body weight. Protein is essential because it also creates a high level of satiety, also know as feeling full. Getting a good dense amount of protein will help you feel fuller longer. It also takes more calories to break down and use than carbohydrates and fat.

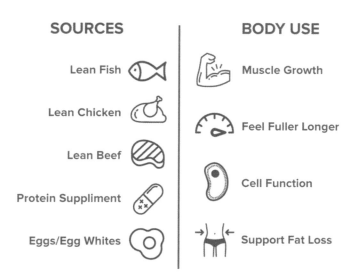

DIETARY PROTEIN USE

SOURCES

Lean Fish

Lean Chicken

Lean Beef

Protein Suppliment

Eggs/Egg Whites

BODY USE

Muscle Growth

Feel Fuller Longer

Cell Function

Support Fat Loss

Carbohydrates are one of the primary energy sources for the body directly. It is used and broken down into basic sugar to be utilized in many body functions. A subset that is very important of carbs is fiber. Fiber is not talked about enough, but it helps with the fluid movement of your intestines for waste and elimination. Where you need to be careful with carbs is its ability to be overeaten. Carbs, especially simple carbs, such as sugar, potatoes, white rice, and grains, can keep you feeling hungry by themselves. One of the reasons why carbs have a bad name is the fact that you can eat and eat and eat them and never feel full. They don't have a high feeling of fullness. It's the reason you don't eat 3-5 chips. You eat an entire bag. Carbs, such as sugar and simple carbohydrates, can spike Insulin in the body and makes you feel hungry again shortly. That's why for the vast majority of people reading this, making sure the carbs you eat are complex is very important. (Sweet potato, brown rice, apples, whole grain pasta)

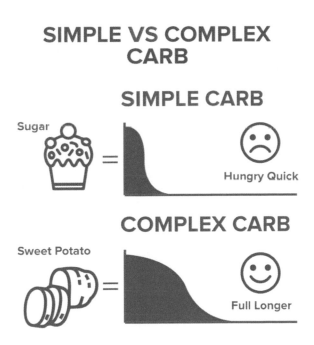

DIETARY CARB USE

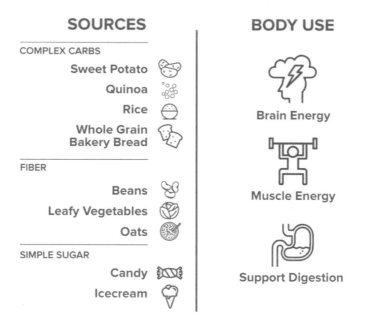

SOURCES

COMPLEX CARBS

Sweet Potato

Quinoa

Rice

Whole Grain
Bakery Bread

FIBER

Beans

Leafy Vegetables

Oats

SIMPLE SUGAR

Candy

Icecream

BODY USE

Brain Energy

Muscle Energy

Support Digestion

Fats also have a very deceiving history. One of the first, and HUGE misconceptions of fats is that fat makes you fat. We had such a war on fat in the past. However, fat has a lot of critical roles in the body. Such as the creation of many hormones. Without fat, in your diet, your hormones can go wild. The big struggle with fat is that since they are 9 calories per gram it is very easy to eat too many total calories because it is so dense in energy. A very positive aspect of fats is it also has very good satiety, meaning it helps you feel fuller longer.

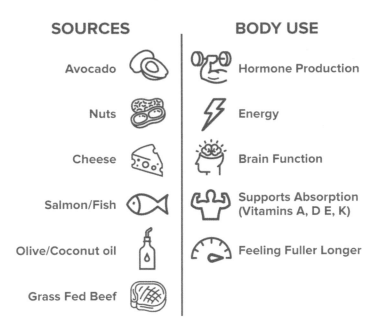

DIETARY FAT USE

SOURCES

Avocado

Nuts

Cheese

Salmon/Fish

Olive/Coconut oil

Grass Fed Beef

BODY USE

Hormone Production

Energy

Brain Function

Supports Absorption
(Vitamins A, D E, K)

Feeling Fuller Longer

Micros

Micronutrients are not talked about heavily during the weight loss process but do play a substantial role. What are micronutrients? They are the other nutrients the body needs to work at its optimal level. The two main sets of micronutrients are Vitamins and minerals. Because vitamins and minerals (with the exception to Vitamin D) cannot be created in the body, they need to be ingested in the diet to prevent disorders of metabolism. There are so many different individual diseases caused by a deficiency in a vitamin or mineral that I won't go into any in specifics, but the list is staggering: atherosclerosis, cancer, osteoporosis.. etc. Due to people's eating habits and how we farm today, the amount of micronutrient deficiencies in the USA is very significant.

What this means to you is simple. I would highly recommend getting on some basic vitamin and mineral supplement. Now, this does not mean you get some Goji berry witchcraft supplement. Just make sure you are getting a clinical dose and accredited source to prove you are getting the dosages it says you are getting. There are minimal problems involved in taking a multivitamin and mineral supplement because at clinical dosages anything that isn't used will just be urinated out.

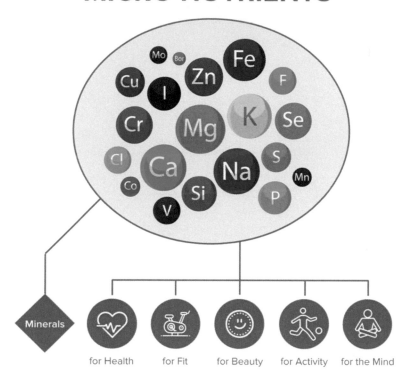

Hydration

We all hear over and over again how we are made up of mostly water. The brain is 73% water. Skin contains 63% water. Even bones are 31% water. Water is by far the most critical factor for life behind oxygen. Our bodies can only go a few days without water before we can have significant problems. The troubling situation happening in the United States is the major problem of not drinking enough water. A study from 2009-2012 showed that 54% of children ages 6-19 years old were not at adequate levels of hydration. (7) This is a very troubling situation sense water is so essential for life.

Dehydration can cause some very interesting symptoms that you may be experiencing right now. Dehydration symptoms: tired, hunger, thirst, headaches. One of the very interesting compensations for dehydration is the holding of fat. With fat having lots of water in it, your body likes to hold on to excess fat. So not only can not drinking enough water make you hungry and tired but it literally can be making you stay fat.

Think about that for you, what are pretty much the top 2 struggles many Americans go through? Tiredness and hunger. We are a group of people in love with coffee and munching. Both of these problems could be actually coming from your bodies desire to have more water.

The standard practice for proper water intake is 10 glasses of water. Personally, I like to do a gallon a day. The way I have also heard to keep proper hydration is half your body weight in ounces. So if you weigh 200 pounds, you should drink at least 100oz in water. For the sake of simplicity, don't take into effect water in foods and other drinks.

A personal experience I had struggled with was tiredness and the love of diet coke. When I came to a conclusion how vital water is to the body, I created the habit of drinking a gallon of water a day. I carried a half a gallon with me. If you don't keep water with you, it makes it hard to stay on track. I made a habit of drinking a half a gallon by noon and half a gallon by the time I went to bed.

A study was done to see how over hydration of 1.5L (50oz) of water a day to a group of obese women over 8 weeks. The results were great. They saw a drop in weight and all the women saw that their appetite went down. (8)

The results of creating that habit were incredible. Let's be honest, when you are drinking a gallon of water a day, you have no desire to drink pop or any other sugary drink. My energy levels went up for sure. When I consistently get my gallon of water in a day, I don't feel hungry as much either. Not to mention, it was one of the first things I changed with my nutritional lifestyle, so it played a huge role in my 150+ weight loss story.

So in conclusion, for proper hydration, I would recommend drinking a minimum of 10 glasses of water a day (80oz). Ideally, I would drink around a gallon, which is 128oz. Get a half a gallon jug, drink one jug by noon and another jug by the time you go to bed.

CHAPTER 8
Intermittent and Extended fasting

Intermittent Fasting and Extended Fasting

One of the hottest topic plans for weight loss of today is Intermittent and extended fasting. Intermittent fasting is based upon the philosophy of feeding windows and fasting windows. First, the long-term logic behind it is the idea, up until about a hundred years ago, it was very typical to go about a day or so without eating. It wasn't until the last 50 years or so this idea that, 3 meals a day is preferred. Or the idea that "breakfast is the most important meal of the day."

For intermittent fasting, there are a few plans. You have two main categories: alternate day fasting and time restrictive eating. In more depth alternate day fasting is exactly how it sounds, you eat every other day. Time restrictive eating is the foundational idea of having an eating window and having a fasted window condensing the time you eat. An 8-hour eating window and 16-hour fasting window is the most common.

What does science say behind it? Why is it effective?

Some of the most significant scientific evidence for intermittent fasting is the ability to blunt appetite. For example, as we have come to learn your body is made to utilize patterns for daily life. We all have that biological clock that helps to wake us when we have a standardized time of waking up. This is the same for eating. Your body will spike hunger signals during the points in time you tend to eat. So, if you were to get the body to condense the window of hunger singles, you wouldn't feel hungry as often and thus make you eat fewer calories, and you lose weight. There tends to be an adjustment period as your body gets used to it. When the body does, you don't feel so hungry throughout the day. (10)

A large myth has been debunked over the last few years that eating small meals throughout the day keeps the metabolism up. This has been proven false. The belief and science behind it were that after you eat there is an increase in energy use in the body to deal with digestion. So the theory was that by eating small meals throughout the day, you will keep your metabolism higher and thus lose more weight. However, the new study shows that the increase in metabolism after a meal is equivalent to the amount of food eaten. Meaning, if you eat 2,000 calories over 10 hours or eat 2,000 calories over 2 hours, the increase in metabolism is the same. (11)

Who would not do well on this plan?

Intermittent fasting is effective for a large set of the population. However, I would highly recommend consulting a doctor for intermittent fasting. If you are on any medications for insulin control or sugar level stabilizers, there is a pretty good chance that you could bottom out your sugar levels in your body, which can cause you to have a low blood sugar reaction. In a non medicated body, it would be able to regulate that, but with medicines influencing the body, it can be dangerous. So if you are looking into doing intermittent fasting, I would consult your doctor first to see how it will affect you.

How would intermittent fasting look?

Take the information from the foundational knowledge. Figure out how many calories you should eat each day and stick your food to that calorie count. Now, your feeding and fasting window can be any 8 hour time you want. You can make it morning to early afternoon or early afternoon to night. Personally, my body has naturally not needed breakfast.

A general overview look at how intermittent fasting (8-16) would look as follows:

A day:

> 6am: wake up, drink 12-18oz of water with or without coffee no sugar or cream

6:30-7:30: gym (cardio or strength training)

12pm: first meal (drink 40-60oz of water by noon)

4pm: second meal

8pm: final dinner (no food after 8pm)

11pm: bedtime, drink 80-120oz of water by the end of the day

Some things to think about when doing intermittent fasting. All calories count for outside of the eating window. So when it comes to adding any type of calorie: add cream to coffee, sugar added to coffee, a little juice. Strictly stick to no calories outside of that window. Another area you should hold a strong resistance to is even synthetic or fake sugars outside of the eating window. Even artificial sugars spike insulin levels in the body. One of the goals of intermittent fasting is to get your insulin levels as low as possible in the body. High insulin levels restrict the use of body fat being used for energy. (12)

Extended Fasting

Extended fasting, as I am referring to, is the consumption of no calories but water for more than 36 hours. "Wait... hold on a sec... I get not eating for 16 hours but 3-5 days?!!?" "No freaking way I could do that"... "I would DIE." Ok, I know this sounds crazy and goes against pretty much EVERYTHING you have been told but hear me out. First, to get how long you really can go fasting; let's look at what we do know scientifically. In 1973, a 27-year-old man weighing in at 457 pounds was eager to make a change. With 457 pounds on his body, that is a lot of stored energy. Under the full supervision of doctors, he did an extended fast. How long do you think he fasted for? 10 days? 30 days? 50 days? 100 days? This man fasted for 382 straight days! He was given vitamin and mineral supplementation but beyond that had no ill side effects and went the rest of his life never going above 200 pounds. Am I telling you to fast for 6 weeks straight? NO!! What I am saying is two things: 1. you can go a lot longer without eating than you think you can and 2. "starvation mode" isn't a real syndrome. Remember, what is fat but stored energy.

I have found extended fasting to be an incredible tool for both weight loss in itself and a mental strengthening exercise. I personally do between 2-4 extended fasts per year. Usually, my fasts run between 3-5 days. During my fasted routine, I drink between 120oz-160oz of water a day. I add 4-6 grams of salt in my water for electrolytes. I drink 2-3 cups of black coffee with no added sugars or creams.

The experience of extended fasting had brought me a lot of great results. During a 5 day fast, I will lose between 8-15 pounds. For which, when I start to eat again I tend to gain back 3-4 pounds. In my experience, day 1-2 tends to be the most struggling days and by day 3 your body has transitioned into Ketosis, utilizing body fat for energy and the body stops releasing hunger signals. After day 3, I don't even feel hungry anymore.

What does the science say? Why is it effective?

This is where I go into more depths that, one size fits all, doesn't work for nutrition. Simply restricting calories or eating healthier doesn't work for certain populations. This is because, especially in the morbidly obese, their hormones are all out of whack. So in the most simple terms, a "reboot" can do wonders for the body. Extended fasting can be a great way to "flip the metabolic switch" and get your body back on track to work correctly. (13,15)

Insulin, we hear this word often. Do you understand what it does? Insulin has many functions, but in the most simple term, it is the hormone used to transfer energy aka sugar into the cells of the body. One of the problems with insulin is it also restricts the metabolism of fat storage. For example, if you are a type 2 diabetic when you use insulin to regulate your sugar levels in your body. It creates an even harder problem to lose weight because high insulin levels make the body hold on to fat even harder.

This is where Intermittent and extended fasts have some serious merit. First, let's look at how most people see calories. Most people see calories as a big bucket in the body. You take in calories and then the body distributes those calories for different stuff. If you eat fewer calories, you will lose weight. The problem with that is the body doesn't really have this 1 size bucket dispersing the calories. It is a two-part system. You have energy that is placed in the liver and muscle called glycogen. You also have the fat storage across your body.

The best way I have heard it explained is the refrigerator vs. freezer comparison. Now, in your fridge, you have glycogen storage. Your refrigerator is easy to get to. If you want an apple, you just have to open the door and grab it. When it comes to body fat, it is like the freezer in the basement. Not so easy to get to. You have to walk downstairs to get something aka energy from fat. However, if your insulin levels and other hormones in the body are too high or too low, it locks the door.

1 PART VS 2 PART

ENERGY SYSTEM

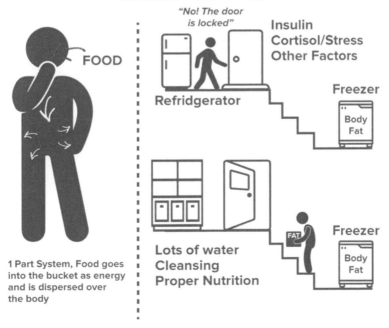

"Flipping of the metabolic switch," a term and mechanism being utilized to change the bodies primary energy source from sugar to fatty-acids aka ketones. I won't go into any detail on how the body does it exactly but what you do need to know is the timeline to "flipping the switch." The "switch," is typically "flipped" between 12-36 hours after food has been eaten. This depends on how much your body stores in glycogen aka "fridge energy." Once the body's storage of sugar is gone, it is forced to switch to using fat as energy. Ketones are then created in the body, from your fat, to be used as energy.

During an extended fast, you should not be doing any strenuous lifting, where you can break down muscle. Such as powerlifting or strength training. You can go on with normal life during a fast. You just should not do any hard activities where you may break down muscle tissue because you don't have any protein to rebuild those tissues. I typically walk 3-5 miles a day during an extended fast.

Do's and Don'ts

First things first, do not do an extended fast without consulting a doctor first. Just like intermittent fasting, if you are on any drugs to help with sugar levels in your body, you will have a big problem in your body running out of sugar before it switches to fat. Resulting in you fainting and hurting yourself.

During an extended fast, I would really focus on getting a gallon of water a day in. With so much flushing happening in the body, it is essential to keep your kidneys clear. A fast longer than 48 hours, I would be adding 3-5 grams of salt to your water a day. You need the salt, or your muscles can get severe cramps.

Do not drink any BCAAs during a fast. Certain BCAAs have an effect on the brain resisting the process of ketosis in the body.

Do your best to stay away from all artificial sugars as they will spike insulin in the body, tricking your brain as if you ate. Holding you back from the best results

Do drink 2-3 cups of black coffee throughout the day.

Your last meal before an extended fast should be low carb and high in fat. Some type of protein and healthy fat. Like a few eggs or chicken with avocado.

Don't allow yourself to use a little bit of hunger pains as an excuse to treat anyone with less respect.

Do take the time to be grateful in the moment. Not for just having the opportunity to make a change, but what it feels like in those first 24-36 hours to know what it feels like not to eat.

CHAPTER 9

KETO

KETO, the new term for an older plan. Many of us have heard about the ATKINS diet of the past. It was a very effective program. Many people saw fantastic results on ATKINS aka a low carb or KETO diet. Many of these terms have become synonymous with each other. In the most straightforward understanding: low-carb, KETO and ATKINS are pretty much the same program. In the most simple explanation. When you lower carbs (lower than 50g a day), the primary energy source of the body, low enough the body has to initiate the fat to take over as the primary source of energy for the body. With also a rise in protein and fats in the body.

The first thing to realize about the KETO plan is, just like any other plan, if you eat a large number of calories above what you burn daily you will not lose weight. So remember, this is not a plan where you can eat your weight in bacon and cream cheese and lose weight. You will have to be conscious of the calories you consume daily.

What does the science say?

The studies have shown many benefits to weight loss and other body functions on KETO. A few of the more well known are: (16)

- Reduction of hunger due to the high protein diet
- Reduction of fat storage and higher fat metabolism
- Efficiency use of energy
- Increase metabolism due to the production of sugar from other processes
- Increase sensitivity to Insulin for type 2 diabetics

Like a lot of the evidence coming from Fasting and intermittent fasting, some people have problems outside of just eating too many calories and not moving their body enough. So KETO becomes a very effective plan because it does many of the same resets that fasting and intermittent fasting do. It helps lower insulin levels in the body opening the door to the more efficient use of body fat as energy. With that added benefit of a high fat and high protein diet makes you feel fuller longer, resulting in you most likely eating fewer calories throughout the day.

KETO vs. Ketoacidosis

Many people hear that KETO is bad for you. Often it gets confused with ketoacidosis. Let's compare the two, so you know the difference. In people with both type 1 and 2 diabetes, when their diabetes is severely uncontrolled, the body makes massive supernatural amounts of ketones. When the ketones get too high of a balance in the blood, it causes the blood to become acidic. This can lead to some very dangerous problems.

However, in KETO, the body is very effective at regulating and controlling the ketone levels in the body. So as your body is at a low level of sugar in the body, it takes the effective and controlled response of creating ketones. Thus making it a therapeutic level for the desired use you want for fat loss. Know that for the vast amount of people out there, KETO is a safe and effective way to lose weight. (17)

KETO vs. Cholesterol

Here is another false understanding of how the body works. We have found this new attack on fat. Fat creates cholesterol and cholesterol kills you. I will never forget sitting down and watching, "What the Health," with my parents. Listening to some OUTRAGEOUS claims.

Now there is plenty of that movie I respect and agree with, like industrialized farming. I am not a fan of how we treat animals in these industrialized systems and all of the chemicals we fill them with. I believe in free range and nonhormonal filled meats. There is a massive difference in the meat from a buck, you killed yourself in the woods. And a steroid filled chicken, that can't even hold itself up because of how big its breasts are.

One of the most absolutely OUTRAGEOUS and OBNOXIOUS claims is how eating one chicken egg is equal to smoking 2 cigarettes. They sit here and bash on cholesterol and fats when it is absolutely unfounded in science. The science has shown in many studies that KETO has actually lowered cholesterol levels and made better levels of HDL and LDL in the body. (18)

What are things to be careful of?

As you decide to use KETO as a program to lose weight, there are a few things you have to be careful of. Just like any other plan, it is smart to consult your doctor to make sure there are no counter-indications for you not to do KETO.

For instance, just like fasting and intermittent fasting, if you are on any insulin or drugs that affect your sugar levels in the body. You will have a severe problem with bottoming out your sugar levels in your body, resulting in you to feel tired or even pass out. So before you do this plan make sure you talk to your doctor about it and it may cause you to check your sugar levels in your body.

As I am a firm believer that there is no: "one size fits all" nutrition plan. The same goes for KETO. If you decide to do KETO, I would recommend that you get a full blood work done after 3 months. It is fascinating how some people's cholesterol levels get better on KETO, and others get worse. The only real way to know is to get blood work done later.

KETO doesn't give you the golden ticket to eat crap either. Like I said before, it doesn't give you the ability just to eat bacon and cream cheese. Knowing healthy fats and healthy proteins are important. Some of my favorite healthy fats are avocado, coconut oil, salmon, almonds, whole eggs.

Heavily restrictive plans such as KETO are a fantastic way to hit your goal. But remember, its not just about hitting your target but SUSTAINING a longterm change. So when you hit your goal, you better have a plan to sustain yourself for the long term. That may mean staying on KETO with 2 CELEBRATION meals a week or that may mean switching it up. The trap that MOST people fall into with heavily restrictive plans is, they lose all the weight but then fall right back into old eating patterns after. You need to be ready and waiting for step 2 after you hit your goal.

KETO CHEAT SHEET

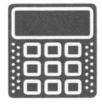

1. CALCULATE DAILY CALORIE INTAKE ON TDEE CALCULATOR:

_____Daily Calorie Intake

2. MACRO BREAKDOWN:

Fat Calories (60-70%) _____ grams

Protein Calories (25-35%) _____ grams

Carbs Calories (0-10%) _____ grams

CHAPTER 10

Carb-Cycling

Carb-cycling is a relatively new nutrition plan that tends to be a hybrid between a few well-known plans. So direct studies and research on it is less prevalent. However, I am a strong proponent of carb-cycling because it is where I got my start, and I find it a very effective plan.

CARB CYCLING CHEAT SHEET

1. Calculate daily calorie intake on TDEE calculator
   _____ Daily calorie intake.

2. Macro Breakdown:

HIGH CARB DAY
Fat Calories (20%)_____grams
Protein Calories (40%)__grams
Carbs Calories (40%)___grams

LOW CARB DAY
Fat Calories (50-70%)_____grams
Protein Calories (40-50%)__grams
Carbs Calories (0 -10%)____grams

3. Weekly Breakdown:

Monday:	Low Carb	Thursday:	Low Carb
Tuesday:	Low Carb	Friday:	High Carb
Wednesday:	High Carb	Saturday:	Low Cab
	Sunday:	High Carb	

Breaking down carb-cycling is pretty self-explanatory. Daily, you cycle between high carb days and low carb days. This becomes the hybrid of different plans and studies. This means there are not many studies done directly on Carb-cycling. However, you can use the KETO and macro counting plans together into what is Carb-Cycling.

Just like any of these plans, you must first find how many calories you must eat daily to lose weight. Once you find your base calorie intake, then you break it down into protein, fat, carb intake. The easiest way to do this is by using the food journal app. This will make sure you track the amount of food you are eating.

The most common of the carb-cycling programs is a 3 day low-carb to 2-day high-carb. Which means for 3 days you are eating high protein mid-fat low-carb, and the other 2 days you eat a high protein low fat mid-carb days. This is allowing you to cycle in more of the foods you enjoy.

CHAPTER 11

Macro Counting

Macro counting is the most longterm sustainable nutrition plan out there, in my opinion. It is the plan where you will be able to live most of your life. What is macro counting? Macro counting is the tracking of your: protein, carbs, and fats. In relation to a calorie goal and macro percentage.

MACRO COUNTING CHEAT SHEET

1. Calculate daily calorie intake on TDEE calculator:
    _____Daily Calorie Intake

2. Macro Breakdown:

Fat Calories (20%)_____grams

Protein Calories (40%)_____grams

Carbs Calories (40%)_____grams

What I find most compelling about macro counting is the ability to be very loose with your plan. You have the ability in the macro counting plan to add small treats during your week and still, fall within your macronutrients and calorie levels.

What you would do to track your macros is to utilize an app, such as MyFitnessPal. This app would track everything you eat daily. One thing that makes macro counting particularly tricky is, to be honest with portion control. Knowing serving sizes for protein, carbs, and fats. Serving sizes can be very deceiving. That's where I would recommend that you weigh your food at the beginning to be able to know what actual portions look like. I have gotten good, from portion controlling in my past, at being able to look at food and be able to judge pretty well the calories in it.

The most normal macro counting program is a 50/30/20 plan. 50% of your calories go to protein. 30% of your calories go to carbs. 20% of your calories go to fats. Now just like I went into many times throughout nutrition plans, you have to find what your sustained calorie level for your body is. You can look it up online by googling TDEE calculator and putting in your information. You don't have to calculate anything yourself. Leverage technology to the best of its ability, by using it to better your life.

From that point, you can put that information into MyFitnessPal and keep track of your food intake. The reason why I do find this plan very sustainable and effective longterm is because of your ability to tweak your plan to have a "cheat meal" without it actually affecting you. For example, if you really want a piece of cheesecake. But you want to stay on track, you can set your day to be very high in protein and low in carb for your first 2 meals. By the end of the day, you can save that 450 calories of sugar and fat for fitting your plan still.

That sounds crazy, right? Be able to eat a piece of cheesecake and still lose weight? That is relatively true with using macro counting correctly. Just like anything else, that's believing your insulin levels are healthy, and body is working correctly.

Remember the foundation of nutrition. All body fat is, is stored energy. So, if you burn more calories than you eat each day, what will happen? Your body must convert stored fat into energy and use it for the body. Thus, making your fat smaller. So by counting your macros, which calculates your calories, you will be able to sustain your ideal body.

The little difference I like to raise is the difference between calorie counting and macro counting. By counting your macros, you understand there is a difference between protein, carbs, and fats. Each has its own primary use in the body. It is more than pure calorie counting and takes into effect what kind of calories they are to be used in the body for primarily. Protein is used for growth and body use. Carbs being used primarily for energy. Fats being used for hormones and other processes.

CHAPTER 12

Workouts

Finally, last but not least, we have working out. Seems so very interesting that I left this last. Not only did I leave this to be the final chapter but I almost didn't even put in this chapter. So very interesting how often I get asked on, "David, what's your workout routine?"… "are you doing drop sets?"… "Are you doing cardio?"… "are you doing powerlifting?".

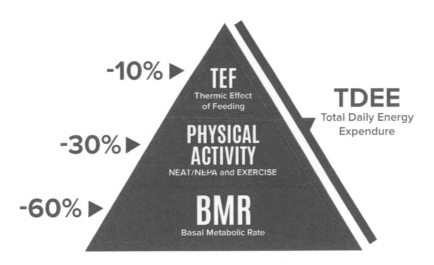

By far the most asked question I get are on what is my workout routine, but in reality, it is one of the most insignificant habits you must do. Weight loss, in it's most straightforward breakdown, is 70% nutrition, 20% working out, 10% supplements and 2000% mindset. Without the proper mindset, you will never stick or even eat right. Without eating right, you will never lose weight. You hear these two areas the most for weight loss, workout routines, and supplementation. In reality, they are the most insignificant areas of your weight loss journey. Just like with money: you can always outspend what you make. You can still out eat what you burn.

Cardio

Now, with that being said. Working out is still a significant piece of the puzzle that can help you, not only lose weight but do it faster and feel better in the process. It is fascinating how for me, I am 255 pounds at this moment but I look better now than I did when I was at my leanest of 235. At the end of the day, it really isn't about the number on the scale but how you physically look and feel. That is where working out has its place.

Countless workout routines come out telling you they are the BEST: CrossFit, HIIT, Cardio, Strength training, Powerlifting, P90X…etc. Before you even start on a program, you must ask yourself, what is my goal? What am I trying to accomplish with this plan? For me, as I said before if you are significantly overweight. I would start with just basic "cardio." Move your body daily. Take 20 minutes to an hour a day to go walk. Maybe biking lightly. It is only about getting the body moving more actively.

Just like in my first year of college. I pushed my body too, and it created too much pain for me. So I quit. The power of momentum is so important. Literally, the first 100 pounds of my weight loss, with working out, inclined walking in the morning and basketball at night.

MOVE, the first step in getting your body in shape is to move it. At the end of the day, as we have learned, burning calories is the primary goal to lose weight. So, if you move the body more and eat less, you will lose weight. You have a few basic types of cardio to choose from: steady state and High-Intensity Interval Training (HIIT). These two are the most basic you hear from today.

Steady state cardio is to sit at a consistent pace over a duration of time. I find steady state a lot more accommodating for most people. By sitting at a constant speed you can learn to pace yourself over a longer time frame burning more calories over time. A few of my favorite steady state cardio choices are: walking, incline walking, jogging, biking, swimming,

CARDIO CHEAT SHEET

Calories Burned Walking 2.5 to 3.5 mph by Miles and Weight (Pace of 17 to 24 Minutes per Mile)						
Weight (lbs)	180	200	220	250	275	300
Mile 1	96	106	117	133	146	160
Mile 2	191	213	234	266	292	319
Mile 3	287	319	351	399	439	479
Mile 4	383	425	468	532	585	638
Mile 5	479	532	585	665	731	798
Mile 6	574	638	702	798	877	957
Mile 7	670	744	819	931	1023	1117
Mile 8	766	850	936	1064	1170	1276

Calories Burned Biking By Weight and Distance					
Weight (lbs)	150	175	200	225	250
Mile 1	48	56	64	71	79
Mile 3	143	167	191	214	238
Mile 5	238	278	318	357	397
Mile 10	476	556	635	714	794
Mile 15	714	833	953	1,072	1,191
Mile 20	953	1,111	1,270	1,429	1,588
Mile 30	1,429	1,667	1,905	2,143	2,381

Incline Walking at 6% Incline By Weight and Distance				
Weight (lbs)	200	240	280	320
Mile 1	184	220	257	294
Mile 2	367	441	514	587
Mile 3	551	661	771	881
Mile 4	734	881	1028	1175

Strength Training

If you believe you are ready for the next level, which is strength training, here is the reason why it is important longterm. One of the most important reasons why you strength train is to put on muscle. What is so important about putting on muscle? I thought I was supposed to lose weight?

Well, let's understand what muscle does. First, it makes you look better haha. Who doesn't want to look better naked? Haha. More importantly, why is that trainers goals are to help you gain lean muscle?

There are 3 main reasons why you want to gain lean muscle:

1. There is a small increase in daily metabolism by gaining lean muscle. It is not as significant as 50 calories per pound that many trainers want you to believe, but if you were to add 10 pounds of lean muscle you would add about 100 calories burned a day. Doesn't sound like much but over a year that's around 3 pounds of fat mass over a year. As long as you hold to the same calories a day.
2. Losing fat and gaining muscle helps you get the toned look better. We have all heard of the "skinny fat" people. Where they are not fat, but they don't look very good because they don't have any muscle mass to make them look leaner and better. That is the same thing as me now. I look better now, 20 pounds heavier than I did before because my muscle to fat is better.
3. Research has made it pretty clear that by adding lean muscle and lowering body fat, you will have a better sensitivity to Insulin. Helping you keep that lean mass stay. (19)

So there are plenty of long-term reasons to want to add lean muscle to your body. It is not as "magical" as many trainers will tell you about 50 calories per pound, but it is still beneficial for you.

When you decide that strength training is important to you, I would recommend that you get a trainer to make sure your form is correct. It is by far the most important thing about strength training. I go to Planet Fitness to workout mostly. It can be fascinating seeing people workout. Often I feel compelled to go up to people doing poor exercises that are on the edge of hurting them. One of the first things I did myself after transitioning from just cardio to strength training was to get a trainer for 2 months to get me the basics. To master anything you must first learn the basics. The basic foundational body movements to strengthen the body.

CHAPTER 13
Final Takeaways and Lessons

So here it is, the compounding of a few hours reading and writing, learning how to make this moment the time where EVERYTHING CHANGES. You DECIDE to TRANSFORM not only your body but also your MIND. SMILE! LAUGH! Close your eyes and VISUALIZE a year from now, seeing what your life will look like committing to EVERYTHING you wrote about earlier. How do you feel? I FEEL FREAKING INCREDIBLE FOR YOU! Knowing this is it! You are a NEW PERSON. You are not your past, and you are REBUILDING YOURSELF.

This book was A LOT of information, so much information that I think it is essential to recap and go into ACTIONABLE STEPS that you NEED to take for this book to be not just entertaining but IMPACTFUL.

ACTIONABLE STEPS

1. Create a desired outcome, "I am so happy and grateful now that..."

2. Find enough REASONS why it is important to you.

3. Chunk down the ultimate goal into something you KNOW without a shadow of a doubt you CAN hit!

4. Create a GOAL/VISION card that you will read out loud 3-5 times a day.

5. Create DAILY minimums or HABITS that will hit that smaller goal.

6. CELEBRATE ANY AND ALL ACCOMPLISHMENTS THAT TAKE YOU CLOSER TO YOUR VISION.

7. Follow me on FaceBook, YouTube and Instagram

After this, I am sure you now have a BURNING DESIRE to TRANSFORM your life. Not just your BODY but also your MIND, your RELATIONSHIPS, and COMMUNITY. Part 1 to this book can be utilized in all six areas of life. PHYSICAL, MENTAL, SPIRITUAL, COMMUNITY, RELATIONSHIPS and MONEY. Those foundational activities and principles can be used to help you in EVERY area of your life. You can see I was pretty quick on the ACTUAL overview of HOW to transform your body on ACTIONABLE STEPS. In the coming months, I will be building out a fully online platform to get in contact with me for a simple one session overview and program setup up to weekly Health Coaching to keep you accountable and on track. I will NEVER be making general plans and programs for the income because NO ONE is GENERIC. So if this is something you would like, you can email me at fitdrock@gmail.com or contact me through the website that I am building out now.

Failure

The F word is one that continues to find strongholds in our mind. The fearing of FAILURE or feeling of being a FAILURE, coming back to previous material. All of our ACTIONS come from one of two areas — the acquiring of PLEASURE or the deterrent of PAIN. However, with CHANGE there will be short term PAIN, the PAIN of DISCIPLINE and PAIN of not being perfect and doing something WRONG.

When it comes down to it, there is only one FAILURE you must not ACCEPT, and that is QUITTING. The ONLY way you don't get your VISION is if you QUIT. I have messed up my nutrition plan more times than I can count. Not just one meal but compounding it into an extended weekend or week and gaining 4,5,6,7+ pounds. What made this last six years different than the previous times was that quitting became TRULY not an option. I made a DECISION that the past was OVER and I was recreating myself. Now does that mean you will be perfect from this point on? Not a

CHANCE. What it does mean is if it takes you 1,2,3,4,5,10+ YEARS. You WILL have your DESIRED outcome. It is INEVITABLE!

The Law of INEVITABLE CERTAINTY

There are three steps into INEVITABLE CERTAINTY. Meaning you can have ANYTHING you DESIRE.

Step 1: Doing the RIGHT THINGS.

- What are the right things?
- You figure those out through MENTORS and MISTAKES.

Step 2: Long Enough

- How long is long enough?
- Until you get your DESIRED OUTCOME

Step 3: CONSISTENTLY

- EVERY DAY, EVERY WEEK, EVERY MONTH, EVERY YEAR.

When you do the RIGHT THINGS, LONG ENOUGH and CONSISTENTLY, you can have ANYTHING you want!

You have learned it's not about the HOW but the WHY. You have created and strong VISION of what you want and WHY it is important to you. You have DESTROYED past beliefs that were hurting you and not helping you. You rebuilt STRONGER BELIEFS that will engage you to take more control over your life. You learned so many different tactics on HOW to be more productive and control your outcome.

Now it is TIME to put it all into USE. By this point, the PROCESS should be ENJOYABLE. Choosing a nutrition plan. Creating a habit of moving the body more. This should now feel more ENJOYABLE and less of a SACRIFICE. I don't feel much SACRIFICE anymore with the DECISIONS

I have made to eat better and move my body more. It is now a way of LIFE. Because this is the VISION I have for myself and what it will take to HAVE and SUSTAIN my body and mind.

I am beyond EXCITED for all of you! How does it FEEL to have DROPPED THE BAGGAGE?

INDEX

1. Your Wish Is Your Command-Youtube

2. Tony Robbins, Awaken The Giant Within.

3. Timothy Wilson, Strangers to Ourselves.

4. The brain,

   http://journals.sagepub.com/doi/abs/10.1177/0956797612473485

5. Pan A, Sun Q, Bernstein AM, et al. Red meat consumption and mortality: results from 2 prospective cohort studies. Arch Intern Med 2012: 172:555.

6. Bellavia A, Larsson SC, Bottai M, et al. Differences in survival associated with processed and with nonprocessed red meat consumption. Am J coin nutr 2014, 100:924.

7. Kenney EL, Long MW, Cradock AL, Gortmaker SL. Prevalence of Inadequate Hydration Among US Children and Disparities by Gender and Race/Ethnicity: National Health and Nutrition Examination Survey, 2009-2012. *Am J Public Health*. 2015;105(8):e113-8.

8. Vij VA, Joshi AS. Effect of excessive water intake on body weight, body mass index, body fat, and appetite of overweight female participants. *J Nat Sci Biol Med*. 2014;5(2):340-4.

9. The Law of Success by Napoleon Hill Pg. 287-318

10. INTERMITTENT FASTS IN THE CORRECTION AND CONTROL OF INTRACTABLE OBESITY. Trans Am Clin Climatol Assoc. 1963;74:121-9.

11. Verboeket-Van De Venne, W., Westerterp, K., & Kester, A. (1993). Effect of the pattern of food intake on human energy metabolism. British Journal of Nutrition, 70(1), 103-115. doi:10.1079/BJN19930108

12. Wilcox G. Insulin and insulin resistance. *Clin Biochem Rev*. 2005;26(2):19-39.